Exposing the Dangers and True Motivations of Conventional Medicine

A Summary of the Most
Commonly Misdiagnosed Illnesses
of Modern Medicine

DR. KEVIN FORD

ISBN: 978-1-4834-2551-1 (sc)
ISBN: 978-1-4834-2552-8 (e)

Library of Congress Control Number: 2015901268

Because of the dynamic nature of the Internet, any web addresses or links contained
in this book may have changed since publication and may no longer be valid. The views
expressed in this work are solely those of the author and do not necessarily reflect the
views of the publisher, and the publisher hereby disclaims any responsibility for them.

Any people depicted in stock imagery provided by Thinkstock are models,
and such images are being used for illustrative purposes only.
Certain stock imagery © Thinkstock.

Lulu Publishing Services rev. date: 1/26/2015

To my father, Joseph Kazakevich, world class
string bass musician and music teacher.

CONTENTS

Manuscript Summary ix

Preface xi

Chapter 1   An Introduction 1

Chapter 2   The Evolution of Modern Healthcare 7

Chapter 3   Pesticides: The Real Pests. 23

Chapter 4   Vaccinations: Information You May Not Know 37

Chapter 5   Dietary Factors: You Are What You Eat. 57

Chapter 6   Sleep Deprivation: Limiting Health and Healing. . .79

Chapter 7   The Air We Breathe 91

Chapter 8   Other Invisible Health Threats: EMR 103

Chapter 9   Making a Change to Pursue Real Health 115

Chapter 10 Food, Diet, and Nutriceuticals 133

Chapter 11 Chelation, Detoxification,
and Hormonal Replacement 149

Chapter 12 Conclusion: The Big Picture 163

Works Cited 167

MANUSCRIPT SUMMARY

Powerlessness, frustration, and insignificance. These are common feelings among Americans when it comes to healthcare today. Costs are exorbitant, access remains poor, and the focus continues to be on services rather than actual health. To make matters worse we are surrounded by an environment saturated in pesticides, herbicides, and chemicals; by foods genetically modified, preserved, and chemically enhanced; and by invisible electromagnetic threats from an explosion of technological devices. Conventional approaches to healthcare with its profit-driven incentives unfortunately react to the problems rather than taking a truly proactive and preventative approach, and our entire industrial and economic system supports its ever-increasing growth despite worsening health outcomes. No wonder feelings of despair abound!

In this book, Dr. Kevin Ford exposes the fallacies and hypocrisies behind conventional medicine today while also providing new directions for improved healthcare. By highlighting personal strategies to augment wellbeing and deter illness, individuals can reclaim the power over their own health and wellness. Through techniques that avoid and minimize exposure to potential health threats and with knowledge of natural dietary, chelation, detoxification, and hormonal therapies, you can once again take charge of your life and longevity without the costs and burdens imposed by traditional healthcare.

PREFACE

Newly released data reports that life expectancy at-birth for the US population reached a record high of 78.8 years in 2012. The US Centers for Disease Control & Prevention (CDC) reports that the age-adjusted death rate for Americans decreased 1.1%, as seniors' life expectancy rose to stand at an additional 19.3 years. Women age 65 and older in 2012 can expect to live another 20.5 years, while men may get around an additional 18 years. The CDC Data Brief attributes the increased life expectancy to an overall greater awareness and implementation of healthy lifestyles.[1]

Lifestyle is a cornerstone of the anti-aging medical approach. University of Zurich (Switzerland) researchers submit that there are four lifestyle choices that can add years to your life. Eva Martin-Diener and colleagues assessed data collected on 16,721 participants aged between 16 and 90 years, enrolled in the Swiss National Cohort (SNC). Identifying the four main risk factors for NCDs as: tobacco smoking, an unhealthy diet, physical inactivity and harmful alcohol consumption, the researchers translated the consequences of an unhealthy lifestyle into numbers. An individual who smokes, drinks

[1] Xu J, Kochanek K, Murphy S, Arias E. "NCHS Data Brief: Mortality in the United States 2012," National Center for Health Statistics (US Centers for Disease Control & Prevention), October 2014; http://www.cdc.gov/nchs/data/databriefs/db168.htm

a lot, is physically inactive and has an unhealthy diet has 2.5 fold higher mortality risk in epidemiological terms than an individual who looks after his/her health. The study authors conclude that: "The combined impact of four behavioural [non-communicable disease] risk factors on survival probability was comparable in size to a 10-year age difference."[2]

Yet, any number of extrinsic factors can potentially ruin a person's best efforts in healthy lifestyle – and thus grossly compromise quality and quantity of life. New challenges that arise from the daunting climate of healthcare today, as well as emerging environmental hazards, are poised to reduce a person's fit, vibrant, vital years.

In *Exposing the Dangers and True Motivations of Conventional Medicine*, Dr. Kevin Kazakevich (Ford) presents insights based on his clinical experiences, to help empower readers and take charge over their personal health and wellness. This book is filled with anti-aging approaches that may help you to extend your years of productive vitality.

Established in 1991 and comprised of 26,000-plus physician, scientist, and health practitioner members from over 120 nations. The American Academy of Anti-Aging Medicine (A4M; www.world-health.net) is dedicated to advancing research and clinical pursuits that enhance the quality, and extend the quantity, of the human lifespan. Every one of our physician members is keenly interested in practical ways to extend the healthy, productive lifespan of their patients.

---

[2] Martin-Diener E, Meyer J, Braun J, Tarnutzer S, Faeh D, Rohrmann S, Martin BW. "The combined effect on survival of four main behavioural risk factors for non-communicable diseases." Prev Med. 2014 Jun 2. pii: S0091-7435(14)00189-3.

As such, the A4M is proud to have Dr. Kevin Kazakevich (Ford), author of this book, as a physician member and Fellow.

Ronald Klatz, M.D., D.O.
President
The American Academy of Anti-Aging Medicine
(A4M; www.worldhealth.net)
October 2014

CHAPTER 1

An Introduction

America is in a healthcare crisis. With such a statement, one might immediately assume the reference relates to rising healthcare costs, limited access to care, and perhaps even controversies surrounding Obamacare. But while these aspects of the nation's healthcare crisis are indeed real, a much larger crisis pertaining to the nation's health exists. This crisis involves how Americans have become socialized into pursuing health and wellness within a healthcare system that has lost its way. It involves a system that is not only failing at the solutions but has likewise become part of the problem. And it involves a system that is no longer able to look at itself in the mirror and see the catastrophe it has become. My hope with this book is to shed some light on this crisis while simultaneously offering a new and effective direction for better health and wellbeing.

Within the last century, dramatic changes have taken place. Industrialization, commercialism, technological explosions, and globalization have all progressed, resulting in a completely new world. While many of these changes have seemingly been beneficial, the environment in which we now find ourselves looks much different than it did decades ago. Global warming is a threat, and pollutants contaminate our air, water, and soil. Foods contain chemicals and pesticide residues that have yet to be defined as safe, and invisible electromagnetic fields surround our every move. To make matters worse the nation's healthcare system contributes to these problems by prescribing billions of dollars of synthetic drugs annually that have a host of adverse effects. It's no wonder that despite these apparent advances of modern-day medicine we find ourselves actually enjoying a reduced quality of life and, for some groups, shortening life spans.

Fortunately we have the power to change this crisis. My father is a perfect example of how a single individual can choose to pursue health in a different manner and escape the threats to health that surround us today. At ninety-seven years of age, my father continuously amazes those he encounters. As a talented musician, he has played the flute, clarinet, and string bass in various symphonies throughout his career, so amazing others is not something new for him. In the 1930s my father even played with Benny Goodman on a regular basis. But today he amazes others due to his physical and mental abilities. For the last ten years my father adopted a different approach to healthcare that did not involve conventional therapies. Instead he chose to pursue an anti-aging regimen that focuses on prevention of disease, preservation of wellness, and natural approaches to health. He is one of the rare nonagenarians (a person in their nineties) to visit the gym several times a week, so the benefits of such a regimen are obvious.

My story is a bit different from my father's. While his story demonstrates how individual effort can overcome the challenges of our current healthcare crises, my story more clearly identifies the specific barriers one may encounter. As a medical physician and an anti-aging specialist, I have seen healthcare from multiple perspectives. I have witnessed the major shortcomings and hypocrisies within traditional medicine while also experiencing the resistance encountered when trying to promote alternative healthcare options. In addition, I have experienced systemic illness related to environmental toxin exposures over my lifetime as well as denials by traditional physicians that such entities exist. And I have realized resolution of my problems through nontraditional therapies that focus on ridding the body of toxins while promoting healthy lifestyles.

As a result of my vast experiences, I appreciate more fully the real underlying motives of mainstream healthcare organizations, and unfortunately these motivations only include better health and wellness as secondary pursuits. But healthcare systems are only one part of the larger crisis. Pharmaceutical corporations, lobbyists, policy makers, licensing boards, chemical manufacturers, agricultural producers, and many other industries are involved in creating a complex web of players with invested interests in sustaining the status quo. It's no wonder different approaches to healthcare that focus on health and wellness as a priority while also dramatically reducing the costs would be received with antagonism.

While this book will expose the foundations and interests of these organizations and entities as they relate to healthcare, the main purpose of the content is to open one's mind to a better approach to health and wellness. In order to accomplish this, greater awareness of the current threats to health must be appreciated. Today our environment contains many perils that didn't exist a century ago, and new hazards are continually being introduced. Unless some knowledge of these threats is gained, avoidance strategies become impossible. For this reason a significant portion of the book describes present-day risks to health and how such exposures can be minimized if not completely avoided.

In addition to an enhanced awareness of health threats and an understanding of avoidance techniques, this book will also describe proactive strategies that will augment health and wellbeing. Unlike conventional medicine, which requires costly medication prescriptions and diagnostic testing, these preventative efforts can be performed on one's own. Better dieting tools, vitamins and supplements, nutriceuticals, exercise regimens, and quality sleep techniques are among the changes one can adopt without relying on health insurance, a scheduled appointment, or medication prescription. With a better understanding of the strategies that naturally promote better health, one becomes empowered to take control of one's own healthcare in a manner that is more effective as well as less expensive.

Though many of the strategies outlined in this book can be implemented independently, some areas may be further advanced through the knowledge and guidance of a specialist. Approaching a conventional physician or other provider will unlikely meet such needs for reasons that will soon be evident. However, specialists do exist who understand and promote preventative healthcare and a more natural approach to wellness. In my experience, anti-aging specialists have a more comprehensive and accurate view of health in this regard and can serve as valuable resources for individuals choosing to take their healthcare into their own hands. The key is to find a health professional who embraces natural therapies and illness prevention as his or her primary focus since this philosophy typically acknowledges the abundance of toxins and threats that exist in today's world.

Without question, numerous books on health and wellness exist, and at any given time several will describe the latest fad, trend, or technique that seeks to help people lose weight, live longer, or become healthier. My intention in writing this book is not to follow in these footsteps of other authors. Instead I wanted to write a book on health that would be timeless. The strategies and the approach to healthcare recommended in this book have existed for millennia because they are based upon natural efforts to preserve wellness and prevent illness. The only thing that has changed involves the environment in which we now live. As long as we have a sound understanding of the health risks present at any given time, the application of the techniques in this book will be consistently effective.

CHAPTER 2

The Evolution of Modern Healthcare

Ask people today what healthcare means to them, and they will likely describe a variety of concepts involving disease and illness, physician evaluation, and diagnostic testing, as well as medicine and surgery. These components of our modern-day healthcare system are taken for granted because of their ubiquitous nature, and very few people consider alternative approaches to health as a result. Interestingly this perspective was not always the case. In fact the development of our modern allopathic approach to healthcare occurred over a relatively brief period of time compared to the more longstanding history of medicine in general. Yet despite its relative infancy, the effects of allopathic medicine dominate everything we perceive when it comes to health. In order to better appreciate the power of this influence, a closer look at the history of healthcare is required.

Organized systems of healthcare actually date back to the fifth millennium BCE as Chinese texts have documented the use of several natural agents in treating illness, preserving health, and prolonging life. Similarly, ancient systems of health management have been noted in Egypt, India, Sri Lanka, and Babylonia.[3] Even in the United States numerous healthcare practices existed prior to the late eighteenth century, demonstrating not only a varied approach to healthcare but also different perceptions of health in general. Only in the last century and a half has our modern system of healthcare developed.[4] Of course this change is perceived as evolving from scientific progress and advancement previously nonexistent, but this assumption fails to appreciate other underlying motivations. After all if such advancements were inherently beneficial, the overall health of the population would be progressively enhanced. Unfortunately this has not been the case.

Today the infant mortality rate within the United States currently ranks thirtieth in the world with 6.9 deaths per one thousand live births, and average life expectancy in the United States is 78.5 years, falling fiftieth among other nations.[5] These results have occurred despite the United States spending more than eight thousand dollars per person on healthcare on average, which reflects 90 percent more than most other industrialized nations globally. In fact, the share of the US economy spent on healthcare is roughly 18 percent, far exceeding any other country.[6] With such poor results despite massive expenditures, how can the nation's healthcare be perceived as the best in the world? This naturally raises the question whether our current healthcare system serves to truly promote health or whether it may serve other purposes and goals. And if the latter reflects a more accurate scenario

---

[3] Plinio, Prioreschi. *A History of Medicine: Primitive and Ancient Medicine*. Omaha, NE: Horatius Press, 1995.

[4] Brown, E. Richard. *Rockefeller Medicine Men: Medicine and Capitalism in America*. Los Angeles, CA: University of California Press, 1979.

[5] N.A. "Healthcare statistics in the United States." HealthPAC Online. Retrieved from http://www.healthpaconline.net/health-care-statistics-in-the-united-states.htm.

[6] Ibid.

then what might be the motivations behind our current healthcare system if better health is not the desired end result? With this in mind, a short history lesson may be helpful.

Historical Systems of Healthcare

Thousands of years ago civilizations did not require people to sit in waiting rooms, have payment options verified, or undergo extensive diagnostic evaluations as a means to encourage good health. Naturally, technological and scientific progress introduced these aspects of healthcare to our modern-day systems. However, ancient times did enjoy systems of healthcare, and the overall benefits particularly in relation to cost of these systems had proven anecdotal results. After all, a system of healthcare had to demonstrate some degree of success in order to stand the test of time. Even today's system of healthcare, despite its relative poor health statistics, shows some positive outcome and effects that substantiate its persistence.

Perhaps the most ancient recorded system of healthcare existed in China; Chinese medicine texts show that some methodical approach to healthcare was pursued as far back as 5000 BCE. Herbal medicines, acupuncture, and therapeutic massage were all utilized as a means to not only cure illness and disease but to also preserve health and prolong life.[7] From a philosophical standpoint the Chinese believed in a causative link between everything existing within the universe and the environment. Thus positive interactions between nature and human beings helped preserve and protect health and life, while negative interactions resulted in the opposite.[8] Through proper diet, lifestyle,

---

[7] Plinio, 1995.
[8] Ibid.

activities, and natural remedies, health could be maximized by allowing the body and mind to be better unified with the universe. The focus was thus on health preservation and maintenance rather than disease intervention and cure.

Herbal remedies have also been noted in healthcare approaches in Babylonia in the second millennium BCE and in India during the first millennium BCE. In fact, sacred Hindu texts dated around 600 BCE demonstrate the synthesis of a variety of traditional herbal practices that sought to protect health and cure disease. According to the Ayurveda, health was perceived as being controlled through human behaviors rather than being predetermined by fate.[9] Therefore health could be influenced through the proper use of diet, natural herbs, and activities proactively to extend life and health. Once again a focus on disease did not lie at the heart of this approach to health. Instead health required an ongoing, active effort to help the mind and body function as normally as possible.

Different perspectives on health systems began to appear in other countries over time. In Egypt an increased attention to anatomy, disease cures, and categories of ailments developed. In fact, the first known surgery was recorded in Egypt in 2750 BCE. In Sri Lanka, despite attention to homeopathic, natural health remedies, a system of hospitals was introduced as a means to encourage health and cure disease. And foundations of Westernized medicine began to evolve in Ancient Rome and Greece as philosophers such as Hippocrates and Aristotle shifted considerations toward human systems and functions.[10] With this shift naturally came an increased attention to aberrancies to normal functioning and health, and identification of disease

---

[9] Ibid.
[10] Ibid.

and pathophysiology began to receive increasing amounts of attention as opposed to health preservation. Cures and remedies began to take precedence over preventative measures of health maintenance.

Allopathic medicine, representing healthcare focused on disease and cures, became most popular in Europe after originating as an established system of medicine in Germany. Bloodletting, leaches, administration of toxins like mercury or lead, and other barbaric interventions were common during the centuries when various plagues swept across the continent. Surgery also became increasingly more common despite the lack of anesthesia and infection control since eliminating the diseased body part was often seen as preferable to other options of treatment and care.[11] During this time a separation between allopathic doctors and homeopathic caregivers began to develop. For example, during the sixteenth century, the well-known prophet Nostradamus served as a plague doctor in France, hired by the public health service to treat Bubonic plague victims while specially trained physicians and surgeons attended to more traditional health issues.[12] Nostradamus was among the first to identify the relationship between better sanitation efforts and reduced infectious spread among the population.[13] This difference of perspective between prevention and intervention epitomized the growing dichotomy between different approaches to healthcare.

This same dichotomy existed in the United States as well during the early years of the nation. In the 1800s competing approaches to healthcare between allopathic and homeopathic doctors were

---

[11] Brown, 1979.

[12] Leoni, Edgar. *Nostradamus and His Prophecies*. Mineola, NY: Dover Publications Inc., 2000.

[13] Smoley, Richard. *The Essential Nostradamus*. New York, NY: Penguin, 2006.

commonplace. Because of the aggressive nature of interventions and the high incidence of complications with medications and surgical treatment, homeopathic physicians using herbal remedies and natural agents actually treated a majority of the people. Rather than pursuing dismemberment or bloodletting, homeopathic physicians sought to use natural, low-cost remedies that helped the body's own ability to maintain health in the face of disease.[14] Unlike allopathic physicians who based their decisions on scientific theory, homeopathic physicians based their practices on empiric observations. Toward the end of the eighteenth century, a healthy competition between allopathic and homeopathic healers existed, but this soon would change.

The Rockefeller Factor

The post-Civil War era represented a watershed event for many changes in the United States, and in some aspects this pertained to healthcare as well. In the latter part of the nineteenth century, progressive industrialization developed, and expansion of markets from the North into the South contributed to capitalist growth. This growth provided the means for a select few to gain tremendous wealth and power through unique opportunities and monopolistic advantages. John D. Rockefeller was one such individual leveraging his early ventures in merchandising into the nation's largest oil-refining operations under Standard Oil Company. Within a short period of time, capitalists such as Rockefeller, Carnegie, and others held a large portion of the nation's wealth, and with this came additional opportunities for influence and power.[15]

---

[14] Brown, 1979.

[15] Brown, 1979.

Healthcare, as previously noted, was poorly organized during this time, and individuals had the choice of pursuing care from either allopathic or homeopathic physicians. The American Medical Association (AMA), which was formed in 1847, increasingly refused to accept homeopathic doctors into their educational and training programs. Instead the AMA adopted scientific theory as its foundation, which strengthened its relationship with pharmaceutical study and the study of human diseases.[16] As a result, Rockefeller and others identified another monopolistic opportunity that could serve their needs moving forward. Specifically, Standard Oil had petrochemical products that could be utilized in the pharmaceutical industry, and increased dependency of the public on such products offered another attentive market for profit.[17] In contrast to homeopathic remedies, which were natural and cheap to acquire, allopathic treatments (and eventually diagnostics) provided a potentially large profit center for industrialized manufacturers.

As the nineteenth century came to a close, several social reforms and trends occurred that facilitated support for allopathic healthcare as well. Social Darwinism supported social views that different classes of individuals offered different potential to society, and thus the fittest would survive while others would not. Therefore class stratification among the population based on talents and abilities was accepted as reasonable.[18] Likewise the Progressive Movement supported advanced education and the development of specialized expertise in promoting social advancements. Scientific evidence and objectivity were viewed as the gold standard by which progress could be made in all fields of

---

[16] Ibid.

[17] Ibid.

[18] Ibid.

study.[19] Both movements encouraged education and acknowledgment of expertise as measures by which quality could be better assessed.

Appreciating this climate, Rockefeller and others developed a strategy by which the American healthcare system as it is known today could be developed. Through large endowments to universities and colleges, and through support of the AMA, Rockefeller and his colleagues served as board of trustee members for many medical educational institutions. In addition political strategies by Rockefeller and others at local and state levels developed strict licensure criteria for practicing physicians.[20] These efforts served two purposes. First, influence on the board directed studies toward allopathic philosophies of healthcare while also restricting the number of potential doctors trained. Secondly, licensure restrictions rapidly eliminated homeopathic physicians from practicing healthcare in society, along with public campaigns that equated homeopathy with quackery.[21] Within a relatively short time period, allopathic healthcare with its inherent focus on disease, drugs, and surgeries became the accepted definition of healthcare services. Through science, technology, and manufacturing, capitalism had created a version of healthcare for the United States guided by the interests of business moguls and corporations.

In essence the development of the US healthcare system evolved under the auspices of philanthropy. Large amounts of financial and resource donations were provided for education, training, and research in the medical field, which in turn yielded incredible discoveries. Advances in our understanding of disease and pathology grew by leaps and bounds throughout the twentieth century as new medicines

---

[19] Ibid.
[20] Ibid.
[21] Ibid.

were designed, new technologies developed, and better surgical techniques adopted. Undoubtedly with each passing decade medical knowledge under the US healthcare system has expanded, allowing new discoveries in both diagnostics and treatments. But despite these advances, overall health among the population has actually declined. In the last few decades obesity has become an epidemic among children and adults alike. And while surgeries involving gastric bypasses and medications to curb appetite have also grown, the overall health of the nation has not improved. Therefore the question arises as to whether such philanthropy was truly beneficial or not.

The pharmaceutical industry, hospitals, and physicians in total have clearly benefited from the persistence of health disorders since the inception of our allopathic healthcare system. But these industries or professions are not the only ones. Initially, as the population accepted the expertise of allopathic physicians as preferable to other types of healthcare, consumers spent their dollars on medications, testing, and hospitalizations according to physician advice. But like many industries in a capitalistic society, some advances became increasingly expensive, exceeding the abilities of many consumers to pay. Once this began to occur, since healthcare is perceived as a right of Americans despite its privileged nature, social programs and private health insurance corporations provided the means by which allopathic healthcare could continue to expand and grow. By distributing the costs among greater numbers of people and by allowing tax dollars to pay for some healthcare services, the healthcare industry continued to enjoy sizable profits.[22] But meanwhile the average quality of health declined despite ever-rising economic costs.

---

[22] Ibid.

Throughout the twentieth century US healthcare has expanded and grown considerably. In the field of diagnostics, an array of radiological tests such as MRI scans, CT scans, and nuclear tests now exist, each at incredible costs to consumers and society as a whole. The amount of money spent by pharmaceutical companies on research and development alludes to the size of revenues often gained from a single popular drug. And despite hospital stay restrictions and legal restrictions on health insurance companies, these corporations continue to stand on stable financial footing. Even during the country's worst recessions, healthcare typically weathers the storm better than any other industry. Yet health in America is far from being the best in the world. Though capitalism has allowed many advances in medicine to be realized under the guidance of philanthropists like John D. Rockefeller, the end result seems to be quite lacking in reaching its primary goal.

An Overview of Current US Healthcare

From a personal perspective, I have experience today's current healthcare system from multiple vantage points. As a child suffering from chronic environmental allergies, I encountered the healthcare system regularly, receiving allergy shots from elementary school through the tenth grade. As a student enrolled in the University of Alabama Birmingham (UAB) medical school, I attended conventional lectures regarding anatomy, pharmacology, and pathophysiology. And at multiple institutions where I performed clinical duties as a medical physician, I experienced firsthand the expected behaviors and practices of a modern-day American physician. But in each instance it was readily apparent that something was lacking. With every encounter the focus of attention was centered on a disease, an illness, or an aberrancy and on how to correct a problem. Though lip service was often given to preventative care and healthy lifestyle, the actual focus of study rarely emphasized these areas of interest.

A perfect example of this preferential focus of education and attention can be highlighted in the time spent on various therapies. Extensive knowledge of medications ranging from pharmacokinetics, chemical structures, side effects, and drug interactions was routinely provided to all medical students and physicians over the course of their training. But the amount of time spent identifying sources of natural antioxidants, the effects of phytonutrients, and nutritional instruction paled in comparison. Likewise the time spent investigating and explaining how regular exercise benefits the body was markedly less when compared to how disease processes affected various organs and resulted in an array of symptoms. With every opportunity the spotlight shone on disease and its effects rather than on health and its preservation. And why not? By constantly shifting attention toward disease, emphasis was placed on medications, surgeries, and other healthcare industry products and services.

When was the last time you went to the doctor's office and left without a medication prescription or an order for some type of testing? Be honest: if you had left without one, would you have felt shortchanged? Each of us has been indoctrinated into our current system of healthcare, and because of this our ability to identify true health-promoting activities is limited. In order to be healthy, we have come to expect the need for some type of medication or surgical therapy. And all the while we fail to actually receive the information we need to be our healthiest.

Let's look at this from an objective perspective. Even within allopathic medicine, sleep has been identified as an important component of our daily lives, promoting better health. Consistently getting adequate hours of sleep allows our immune system to function more effectively, reduces cognitive errors, promotes healthy moods and attitudes, and has been linked to greater longevity. However, one of the most consistent practices among medical education and residency programs involves grueling schedules that limit and interrupt sleep for physicians in training. If conventional medicine considered health-promoting practices as a priority, one would assume these would naturally be incorporated into its policies and procedures.

The same can be said about medications and surgeries in comparison to proactive health-promotion efforts. Without questions, medications offer many benefits to patients for a variety of diseases. Likewise surgery offers many patients cures and relief for an array of ailments. But no matter how advanced these allopathic therapies become, they will never be as effective as preventing disease in the first place. Despite scientific research and clinical trials, these therapies will continue to have negative side effects on health from time to time due to an incomplete knowledge of their effects on the human body. How many times has a new medication been released for use only to be removed from the market a few years later when serious adverse effects are identified? Many attorneys have benefitted greatly from these circumstances.

Conventional healthcare has encouraged the development of synthetic chemicals by large pharmaceutical companies for the management of disease more than they have for the cure. Among elderly individuals, more than 40 percent take five or more medications on a daily basis.[23] Additionally, the knowledge among pharmacists and

---

[23] Brody, Jane E. "Too many pills for aging patients." *The New York Times*, April 16, 2012. Retrieved from http://well.blogs.nytimes.com/2012/04/16/too-many-pills-for-aging-patients/?_r=0.

physicians about the interactions among this number of drugs and their combined effect on the human body remains unknown in many instances. According to the Centers for Disease Control (CDC), over 700,000 adverse drug events (ADEs) result in emergency room visits annually in the United States, while ADEs cause 120,000 yearly hospitalizations. Estimations of the cost of these adverse events total more than $3.5 billion.[24] Thus conventional healthcare not only fails to correct the underlying health problem and promote healthy behaviors, but it also contributes to the decline in the overall health of the nation while also adding to its financial costs.

While the current medical healthcare system in the United States is failing due to its focus on allopathic approaches to health only, many other industries are also contributing to the nation's health crises. For decades now pesticides and insecticides have been used in the agricultural industries, contaminating livestock and food products that we consume. Genetically modified foods also pose health risks to us, although the scope of their ill health effects remains poorly studied. Chemical compounds and heavy metals added to foods, medicines, and vaccines as preservatives also present toxins to the human body, which can affect health. And environmental changes in air and water quality have notably exposed populations to detrimental changes such as rising carbon dioxide levels, reduced oxygen levels, volatile organic compounds (VOCs), and flame-retardant chemicals. Even the exponential increase in electromagnetic radiation in the atmosphere has been shown to negatively affect hormonal balance and cognitive function.

Unlike conventional medicine, homeopathic healthcare primarily

---

[24] Centers for Disease Control (CDC). "Medication Safety Basics." *CDC.gov.* Retrieved from http://www.cdc.gov/medicationsafety/basics.html.

seeks to identify the course of the health problem while also encouraging health-promoting behaviors. Rather than developing synthetic chemicals, natural and herbal agents are preferentially used. Instead of counteracting the effects of food and environmental toxins by treating secondary side effects, detoxification efforts are attempted while avoiding further toxin exposure. And rather than providing additional ways to treat disease in the body, ways to augment the body's natural defense and health mechanisms are pursued in a collaborative approach. The current US healthcare system ranks low in the world for a reason, and this reason is a reflection of the system's approach to disease, illness, and health. Perhaps the time for a long, hard look at the actual premises upon which the system has been based for more than a century is warranted.

Putting It All Together

To appreciate the American system of healthcare and its limitations, a broader perspective of health in general is needed. For millennia cultures and societies have utilized a variety of methods to promote, maintain, and achieve better health through natural strategies of care. While technological and scientific advances have certainly deepened our understanding of the human body and its physiology, reliance on these areas for healthcare is not required. In fact, despite these remarkable discoveries and advances, nothing has yet to compare to the human body's natural abilities to repair itself from disease and injury or protect itself from harm. As a result allopathic medicine should be an adjunctive component of healthcare, but instead it has become both our starting and ending points by which health is currently measured.

These observations regarding allopathic healthcare are not meant to indict our healthcare system in total. However, understanding how capitalist and commercial interests help shape the US healthcare system is important so that motivations and incentives can be better understood. Many stakeholders within the healthcare industry enjoy benefits when disease is perpetuated and when utilization of the healthcare system is high. Pharmaceutical companies, health insurance corporations, physicians, hospitals, medical equipment companies, and many more have an invested interest in assessing and treating injury, illness, and disease. In contrast, few stakeholders other than society at large have strong incentives to prevent disease and maintain health. Natural and herbal remedies offer little opportunities for profit, and prevention efforts fail to demand ongoing needs for services and products. Despite the advantages greater health would bring to us as a nation, individual corporations and entities do not have strong incentives to pursue such a healthcare system as a whole.

To consider this perspective from an even deeper viewpoint, secondary motives in addition to profits may also influence current strategies in American healthcare. The ability of individuals and corporations to maintain power positions through specific healthcare practices has been proposed as another reason allopathic and conventional care is preferred. For example, population control and eugenics have been suggested by some analysts as underlying motives for some vaccination programs and other therapies.[25] While this may sound like a conspiracy theory of sorts, manipulation of health and other factors such as economic status and political power has occurred

---

[25] Taylor, Daniel. "Vaccinate the World: Gates, Rockefeller Seek Global Population Reduction." *Global Research*. September 7, 2010.

throughout history as a means to attain the desired goals of a powerful few.

Though underlying motives for today's current healthcare system may be debatable, the functional ability of US healthcare to promote and preserve health is certainly lacking in comparison to other nations throughout the world. Medical professionals and the public lack awareness of toxic exposures in the environment and in our food sources, and knowledge of how to avoid and rid the body of these substances is limited among most healthcare providers. Unfortunately this reflects a substantial shortcoming of conventional medicine. Since the likelihood that allopathic healthcare will suddenly incorporate anti-aging and homeopathic strategies into its paradigm is small, we must educate ourselves in these topics of interest. By empowering ourselves with deeper knowledge and understanding of health, we can make more informed decisions about how we choose to approach healthcare in general.

CHAPTER 3

Pesticides: The Real Pests

According to the World Health Organization, approximately three million agricultural workers are poisoned by pesticides each year; of these, roughly eighteen thousand succumb to their illness annually.[26] Considering that the use of pesticides, insecticides, and herbicides is to enhance the quality of human life through better agricultural production, these figures are quite astounding. But pesticide use in the United States is big business. Approximately $20 billion is spent on pesticides worldwide each year. For every dollar spent on pesticides, crop yields and subsequent profits are increased four times this expense.[27] This simple fact makes it clear why human health and safety may not always be a top priority when pesticide use is being considered.

Pesticides, which include a large number of chemicals aimed to inhibit or destroy insects, molds, fungi, and other pests, consist of an array of chemicals that interfere with normal cellular or metabolic

---

[26] Miller, G. Tyler Jr., and Scott E. Spoolman. *Sustaining the Earth*. Belmont, CA: Brooks/Cole Cengage Learning, 2010.

[27] Pimentel, David, Herbert Acquay, Michael Biltonen, P. Rice, M. Silva, J. Nelson, V. Lipner, S. Giordano, A. Horowitz, and M. D'amore. "Environmental and economic costs of pesticide use." *BioScience* 42, no. 10 (1992): 750-760.

functions. To a degree these chemical effects are often tailored to the specific organism targeted by the pesticide, but effects on other organisms are inevitable. As a result persistence of these chemicals in our environment or contamination from residues of these materials in foods, soil, and water poses threats to our own normal functioning. Repeatedly, negative health effects such as cancers, hormonal dysfunctions, birth defects, and developmental problems have been associated with pesticide exposure among human populations, but many times these problems have only been identified after large numbers of people have been affected.[28] Despite the restriction of some pesticide agents today, an increasing number of pesticides are being produced and applied with a relatively small degree of awareness of their long-term potential for poor health effects.

In this chapter we will explore both the past and present use of pesticides in the United States and the current regulatory process involved in overseeing pesticide use. These discoveries will highlight the difficulty in determining the relative safety of pesticides and also demonstrate the common occurrence of side effects from these agents. As the demand for foodstuffs increases to meet a growing population, enhanced agricultural production efficiency is required. Both pesticides and genetic medication of foods seek to meet this demand but in the process raise serious issues about health, safety, and underlying motivations.

---

[28] Alavanja, Michael CR, Jane A. Hoppin, and Freya Kamel. "Health Effects of Chronic Pesticide Exposure: Cancer and Neurotoxicity* 3." *Annual. Rev. Public Health* 25 (2004): 155-197.

Pesticides and the US Regulatory Process

According to the Stockholm Convention on Persistent Organic Pollutants, nine of the twelve most dangerous organic chemicals in the world are pesticides.[29] Pesticides have been utilized for crop protection as well as for other purposes for centuries. In fact DDT, which is a well-known pesticide associated with numerous health effects, was invented in the mid-nineteenth century. Originally used to reduce insect populations causing diseases like malaria, DDT was later used to control a variety of insects and other pests in agricultural settings. Of course DDT was later found to result in numerous endocrine, developmental, and carcinogenic problems among human populations and has since been banned for use.[30] But the persistence of DDT in fatty tissues of fish and other animals served to cause health problems long after its use was discontinued.

In the United States, the Environmental Protection Agency (EPA) regulates pesticide use and determines minimal chemical residues standards for each substance in relation to its usage. Likewise pesticide manufacturers are required to perform a variety of tests and studies examining toxicology, residues, and side effects from exposure before a pesticide is approved for public use.[31] This scientific approach, which coincides with allopathic philosophy, seems reasonable as a means to determine chemical safety; however, a major problem

---

[29] Chemicals, U.N.E.P. "Ridding the world of POPs: A guide to the Stockholm Convention on Persistent Organic Pollutants, the Secretariat of the Stockholm Convention and UNEP's Information Unit for Conventions." (2005).

[30] Ecobichon, Donald J., and Robert M. Joy. *Pesticides and neurological diseases*. Boca Raton, FL: CRC Press, 1993.

[31] EPA. "Pesticides and Public Health." 2008. Retrieved from http://www.epa.gov/pesticides/health/public.htm#regulation.

in the process exists. Chemical manufacturers are only required to test pesticides in isolation during these studies, yet these chemicals are combined with a variety of other chemical agents either through administration or after application. Evaluation of any synergistic effects these chemicals may cause to health remains untested prior to regulatory approval.

Pesticides come in different categories based on their chemical structures. Common pesticides include organophosphates, carbamates, organochlorines, pyrethroids, and sulfonylureas. Of these categories the organochlorines are perhaps the most notorious for causing long-lasting effects because of their tendency to be stored within fatty tissues. As a result, their persistence in the environment and within the human body is much longer. For example, chlordane, which is an organochlorine pesticide, has a half-life of ten to twenty years.[32] This means any given amount of the chemical requires this duration of time to be reduced in half. Overall, the elimination of any chemical is defined by approximately five half-lives. So for chlordane, its persistence in the environment can last anywhere from fifty to one hundred years after use.

Chlordane, like DDT, which is also an organochlorine, was restricted from use and taken off the market by the EPA in 1988 due to its noted toxicity. Prior to 1983 chlordane was commonly used on citrus and corn crops as a pesticide, and prior to 1988 chlordane was a popular agent used against termites as well as other household insects.[33] As misfortune would have it, I was performing my clinical rotations in my third year of medical school in Tuscaloosa, Alabama, in 1983, and the building in which we stayed as students suffered a

---

[32] Ecobichon and Joy, 1993.
[33] Ibid.

severe infestation of cockroaches. Insecticide was repeatedly sprayed and sprayed in an effort to rid the building of these pests, and due to the age of the structure and its heavy paint-sealed windows, the ability to ventilate the building with fresh air was very limited. During this time I suffered from extreme fatigue, poor concentration, reduced memory capacity, and intermittent anxiety. I can only suspect the pesticides being used contained chlordane and that my complaints were indeed related.

While chlordane might not have been the only culprit involved in causing my symptoms, I later found out my exposure to chlordane had been significant. As a result of testing performed in 2004, I found that residual chlordane levels remained in my body stored within fatty tissues. In other words chlordane remained in my body despite my being exposed to the chemical twenty years prior. Given the fact that chlordane was also used to treat citrus and corn crops prior to 1983, ingestion of these foods or meats from animals given corn-based feed prior to this date likely reflected another source of contamination for me. Regardless, a significant part of the problem associated with pesticide exposure in relation to health involves the delayed effects these chemicals can have on the human body and their capacity to hang around for years after exposure. Relying on scientific studies to reveal such health effects is understandably limited due to the delayed amount of time between cause and effect, and therefore studies suggesting chemical safety may often fail to tell the entire truth.

DDT and chlordane are not the only notable pesticides associated with failed safety protections in the United States. Most everyone is familiar with the pesticide Agent Orange, which was utilized in massive quantities during the Vietnam War as a defoliate. This herbicide developed by the US Department of Defense in conjunction with

Montsano Corporation and Dow Chemical aimed to eliminate the dense foliage of South Vietnam being used as military cover by guerilla forces. Millions of gallons of Agent Orange were dropped over Vietnam, mixed with jet fuel, in amounts far exceeding recommended administrations. In final estimates, approximately an eighth of the terrain in South Vietnam was exposed to this chemical, resulting in widespread exposure to civilians, military, and livestock.[34]

While Agent Orange itself contains two herbicide compounds with their own inherent toxicities, contamination of the product with another potent chemical named TCDD occurred during administrations during the war, causing more profound effects on human health. Some estimates ascribe half a million birth defects in children to these combinations of chemicals between 1961 and 1971, when Agent Orange was used, and nearly the same number of adult deaths and disabilities occurred as a result of Agent Orange as well.[35] Similarly, many US military personnel exposed to Agent Orange experienced negative health complaints after the war, but the number actually acknowledged as having "Agent Orange Syndrome" represented a small fraction of those voicing symptoms. Despite policies today that speak strongly against the use of chemical warfare, the statistics associated with Agent Orange demonstrate how pesticide practice often ignores safety considerations and subsequently the aftermath created.

---

[34] Stellman, Jeanne Mager, Steven D. Stellman, Richard Christian, Tracy Weber, and Carrie Tomasallo. "The extent and patterns of usage of Agent Orange and other herbicides in Vietnam." *Nature* 422, no. 6933 (2003): 681-687.

[35] York, Geoffrey, and Hayley Mick. "Last Ghost of the Vietnam War." *The Globe and Mail*. Toronto, ON, Canada: Phillip Crawley (2008).

Environmental Considerations with Pesticides

Because different chemicals used as pesticides exhibit different mechanisms of action, their effects on human and environmental health vary from agent to agent. However, some common concerns exist among all pesticides in how they interact with our environment and with our bodies over time. For example, two pesticides may have different degrees of toxicity, but the extent to which each spreads through the atmosphere and persists in the environment may result in both having relatively equal concerns to long-term health. For this reason, short-term and long-term effects of pesticides are important. Appreciating this fact supports the need for more comprehensive efforts toward health and safety measures in relation to pesticide use. A scientific study of a single agent in a laboratory setting over a few years is unlikely to reveal the entire picture when it comes to pesticide effects on our health.

One important health concern regarding pesticides in general involves the exposure of areas that are not targeted for administration. Pesticide drift is defined as the tendency for pesticides to travel in particles through the air to areas remote from their intended administration. For example, chlordane has been found as far away as the Arctic Circle, where it has never been administered.[36] With pesticide drift, chemical particles evaporate and enter the earth's atmosphere, where they travel hundreds to thousands of miles from their site of

---

[36] Bidleman, Terry F., Lisa M.M. Jantunen, Paul A. Helm, Eva Brorström-Lundén, and Sirkka Juntto. "Chlordane enantiomers and temporal trends of chlordane isomers in Arctic air." *Environmental Science & Technology* 36, no. 4 (2002): 539-544.

application. Eventually these same particles fall back to the earth in the form of precipitation and contaminate areas that were never intended to be exposed to such chemicals.

Water and soil pollution from applied pesticides represent other common problems. Chemicals applied to agricultural fields presume isolated and limited administration, but the residual amounts of these chemicals in the soil can accumulate over time and increase the degree of pesticide exposure to crops grown in these fields. If different pesticides are used over several years, chemical interactions among these residues may pose unknown threats to human health from the resultant food products grown. Likewise livestock feeding in these same areas may also become adversely affected from chemicals in the ground.[37] These scenarios are difficult to simulate and study in the laboratory, and because of this our knowledge of the long-reaching effects of soil pollution is limited.

Water pollution reflects a similar concern. In rural areas, rain runoff from fields treated with pesticides can enter ponds, streams, rivers, and lakes, which in turn must be treated before the water can be safely used by individuals. In some instances livestock water supplies are inadequately treated, and these animals are exposed to increasing concentrations of pesticides over time. Fish living in such freshwater sources can also become affected by pesticide chemicals as can animals that eat the fish naturally or drink from these freshwater areas.[38] If these fish or animals are utilized as food for human populations, this represents another way by which pesticides can affect human health unknowingly.

---

[37] Miller and Spoolman, 2010.
[38] Ibid.

Biological magnification describes this process where chemicals within the environment gradually become more concentrated and prevalent within the environment over time as a result of natural occurrences. Water contaminated by chemical pollution results in fish with increased concentration of chemicals. Mammals that eat these fish then become contaminated as well with chemical levels increasing in their bodies as the number of fish consumed increases. Through the food chain, including humans, all species involved gradually accumulate progressive levels of these toxins within their biological systems. For pesticides like chlordane that are easily stored in fatty tissues and have prolonged half-lives, their ability to persist in the environment and in numerous species for years is astounding.

From a larger perspective, pesticides also affect the environment through negative effects on biodiversity. By destroying habitats and specific insects, plants, or other living entities, pesticides alter the natural course of biological interactions, resulting in imbalances and shifts in ecology. In any given situation these ecological shifts may restrict specific resources needed for good health or pose new threats to healthy living.[39] Though targeted use of pesticides is attempted, rarely are these attempts successful. Some studies have demonstrated that 98 percent of all insecticides and 95 percent of all herbicides reach areas that were never intended to be exposed to these chemicals.[40] Unless pesticides can be studied more completely and for much longer periods of time, their safety in relation to both human and environmental health remain at the very least questionable and at the most seriously concerning.

---

[39] Ibid.
[40] Ibid.

Specific Health Effects Related to Pesticides

While pesticides come in a variety of classes and categories, their effects on human health can be grouped into three main areas. The first involves neurological health effects as many pesticides specifically interfere with nerve function and are considered neurotoxins.[41] For example, DDT causes sodium channels on nerve cell membranes to remain open, resulting in over-excitation of nerve cells and spasm. Eventually this results in nerve cell death. Other pesticides commonly interfere with chemicals that allow nerve cells to communicate with one another. For instance, both organophosphates and carbamates interfere with the neurotransmitter acetylcholine, causing nervous system dysfunction and secondary muscle paralysis.[42] Because of this common mechanism of action of many pesticides, health effects involving the brain and nervous system are common complaints among individuals exposed. Symptoms can range from tingling numbness, headaches, memory loss, concentration difficulty, fatigue, muscles weakness, and insomnia to more serious problems such as muscular dysfunction, incoordination, psychological manifestations, and visual problems.

The second common health effects related to pesticides involve genetic damage to cells within the body. In adults, cellular damage to DNA caused by pesticide chemicals can result in the development of cancer cells. Tissues with rapid cellular turnover are particularly vulnerable to pesticide effects in causing malignancies. As a result testicular cancer, leukemia, lymphoma, and colon cancer have been associated with many pesticides. Breast cancer, prostate cancer, and

---

[41] Ecobichon and Joy, 1993.
[42] Ibid.

lung cancer are less common health effects.[43] Damage to DNA structures also results in health effects involving child development. And increases in the number of miscarriages and stillbirths have been associated with pesticide toxicity in addition to birth defects involving numerous organ systems. In each of these instances, the underlying damage to genetic DNA material within cells results in changes causing abnormalities to evolve.

The third category of health effects related to pesticide exposure pertains to the endocrine or hormonal systems of the body. Interference of hormonal regulation can result in widespread health effects. For example, pesticides have been commonly associated with fertility and reproductive problems.[44] In part these effects may be due to genetic damage to reproductive cells, but similarly hormonal imbalances resulting from pesticide exposure create poor environments for reproduction to proceed. Some pesticides like DDT and chlordane are known to affect endocrine systems. Thyroid dysfunction and menstrual irregularities have been associated with DDT exposure, while chlordane has been linked to higher rates of diabetes mellitus.[45] Health requires proper hormonal balance, as will be discussed later in the book, and pesticides can cause this balance to be negatively affected, resulting in ill health effects.

From laboratory testing performed later in life, I now realize many of my complaints during my own medical training were due to exposure to pesticides. As mentioned, residual amounts of chlordane persisted in my body more than twenty years after exposure to the

[43] Alavanja, Hoppin, and Kamel, 2004.

[44] Sanborn, M., K. J. Kerr, L. H. Sanin, D. C. Cole, K. L. Bassil, and C. Vakil. "Non-cancer health effects of pesticides: Systematic review and implications for family doctors." *Canadian Family Physician* 53, no. 10 (2007): 1712-1720.

[45] Miller and Spoolman, 2010.

chemical. And my tissue levels of tin exceeded acceptable amounts by fortyfold. The organic form of tin is found in plastics, paints, and even toothpastes (as stannous fluoride), but tin is also a component in many pesticides. Exposure to tin can occur through a variety of ways not only involving ingestion and respiration but also through absorption directly through the skin. Like chlordane, tin is extremely persistent in the environment in its organic form, being resistant to degradation and breakdown. Based on these chemical levels in my body and my array of symptoms, I have little doubt pesticides played a significant role in the decline of my health.

Prior to 1980 my ability to function academically as well as socially was superb. I was granted a full scholarship to the University of Arizona, and I performed as a professional cellist in the Alabama Symphony after this. Even in the years to follow, I consistently scored exceptionally well on standardized medical tests, often ranking in the ninety-fifth percentile among US medical students. But despite this a variety of symptoms began to plague me and my ability to perform. Declines in concentration, attention, and short-term memory developed, and irritability and insomnia were often present. My behaviors were often described as chaotic, distracted, and fragmented with a lack of focus. Interpersonal relations increasingly became a challenge. If I had only realized the source of my problems then, avoidance of further exposure to toxins and detoxification efforts could have been pursued much earlier.

My situation, however, is not an uncommon one. Even today pesticides being used are likely affecting the health of individuals and the environment without knowledge of the effects. Due to biological magnification, delayed effects, chemical persistence, and synergistic effects among an array of chemicals, the ability to determine pesticide safety is nearly impossible through the limitations of scientific study. Numerous alternatives to this dilemma exist fortunately. The use of naturally occurring biological pest controls such as pheromones and bacterial pesticides have shown success. Agricultural techniques such as steaming the soil, rotating crops, planting numerous crops in a single area, and strategic geographic selection all provide pest control without introducing potentially harmful chemicals.[46] But these efforts rob large chemical manufacturers of profits and may not yield the same magnitude of crops for sale when compared to the use of pesticides. Once again the decision to trade profits for health seems to be at the root of the problem.

If we desire to truly improve our health, healthcare systems must pay attention to the underlying cause of many health conditions rather than symptomatically treating complaints as they occur. History has provided ample evidence that pesticides are a cause of many health disorders, but this realization fails to be appreciated until years and sometimes decades after exposure. Preserving health drops down on the list of priorities when it comes to pesticide use. Marginal safety guidelines are implemented as regulatory efforts, and approved pesticide use continues as a means to fuel larger industries in the agricultural and chemical manufacturing areas. Likewise conventional medicine has failed to investigate these foreign environmental agents adequately as the cause of many genetic, endocrine, nervous system, and cancer-related conditions. The time for a change in the approach to healthcare has come. Greater awareness of the harmful effects of pesticides represents the first step, and a change in healthcare perspective is the second.

---

[46] Ibid.

CHAPTER 4

Vaccinations: Information You May Not Know

Vaccinations are a part of our lives and have been since the middle of the twentieth century. Illnesses such as smallpox and poliovirus provided opportunities for the use of vaccinations in deterring disease and protecting populations from serious health concerns, including death. For these disorders, the occurrence of substantial health effects related to these diseases warranted aggressive considerations. However, the development of these vaccinations paved the way for many subsequent immunizations, and their benefit-risk profiles are not nearly as impressive as their predecessors. In fact, significant evidence supports that many harmful effects related to subsequent vaccines exist.[47] But despite this evidence widespread support for mandatory vaccinations remains popular.

In the United States today less than 1 percent of children fail to

---

[47] Moritz, Andreas. *Vaccine-Nation: Poisoning the Population, One Shot at a Time.* Ener-Chi Wellness Center, 2011.

receive any vaccination whatsoever.[48] The vast majority instead receives numerous injections of immune antigens of various bacteria and viruses with the presumed intention of stimulating the child's immune system to ward off disease. But in the process contaminants and preservatives associated with these vaccines gain access to our bodies. The effects from these vaccinations on our immune systems are likewise not thoroughly understood. This is particularly true for children under six years of age, whose immune systems are still developing.[49] Regardless, with each passing decade the number of vaccinations required or encouraged slowly increases, raising the cumulative total of foreign antigens received. One naturally must wonder how individuals survived centuries ago without such interventions.

On the surface the use of vaccinations by conventional medicine seems to be a step in the right direction, striving to invest in preventative measures to avert disease and promote health. However, a more detailed examination shows vaccinations serve capitalistic needs of major pharmaceutical companies as well as the healthcare industry in general. And the real benefits from these agents are questionable, especially in the face of rising health disorders related to impaired neurological development, altered immune system functioning, and the appearance new infectious organisms. From this perspective vaccinations are simply another way by which conventional medicine and outside interests serve self-fulfilling needs while real health is neglected.

---

[48] Beasley, David. "Survey shows more U.S. children getting vaccines." Reuters. Sept. 1, 2011. Retrieved from http://www.reuters.com/article/2011/09/01/usa-vaccines-idUSN1E7801L020110901.

[49] Moritz, 2011.

Vaccinations and Their Advancement over Time

The development of vaccines dates back to as early as the eighteenth century, when cowpox virus was used to infect some individuals as a means to deter smallpox.[50] However, the first mandatory vaccine policy occurred in the United Kingdom in 1853, when smallpox vaccinations were required for all individuals. Subsequently, the appearance and spread of specific diseases triggered greater interest and development of vaccines as solutions to public health problems.[51] For example, the increase in poliovirus infections prompted greater research into the development of a polio vaccine in the 1950s, and increasing outbreaks of congenital rubella in the late 1960s led to the creation of the MMR vaccine (measles, mumps, and rubella).[52] Thus while vaccinations and their effects on the immune system have been appreciating for some time, vaccine development (just like conventional medicine) advanced in reaction to existing health disorders.

The real revolution in vaccine development occurred in the middle of the twentieth century. After Jonas Salk developed the injectable vaccine for polio, researchers such as Sabin and Hilleman focused their efforts on vaccine development as well at the Merck Pharmaceutical Company. Maurice Hilleman was particularly noteworthy in his endeavors, creating fourteen different vaccines during his career in public administration. Vaccines against mumps, measles, rubella, diphtheria, pertussis, and tetanus were among the more well-known vaccines developed by Merck during Hilleman's tenure,

---

[50] Riedel, Stefan. "Edward Jenner and the history of smallpox and vaccination." *Proceedings (Baylor University Medical Center)*. Jan. 2005; 18(1): 21-25.
[51] Ibid.
[52] Ibid.

and mandatory vaccinations soon became the standard for any child attending public schools.[53] The initial administration of the polio vaccine as well as these other childhood vaccinations were heralded as medical breakthroughs with media reports glamorizing their effects and the lack of side effects. This positive feedback encouraged greater efforts in vaccine development, leading to an ever-increasing number of vaccination administrations required for children. As of today the Centers for Disease Control recommends children during their first year of age receive fourteen different vaccinations with many of these given in multiple doses. In fact by twelve months, most children have received twenty-three vaccination injections in total.[54]

Of course the number of injections is of little significance since the risks are so minimal, right? Interestingly the National Childhood Vaccine Injury Act passed in 1986 developed a Vaccine Adverse Event Reporting System based on increasing complaints among parents criticizing mandatory vaccination schedules. Since that time more than 350,000 complaints have been reported, and independent reviews of these complaints identify 13 percent as being serious.[55] The current stance by the scientific community holds that the benefits of vaccines outweigh their risks or side effects, but the need for such protection from infectious diseases is questionable. For example, the occurrence of hepatitis B in children in the United States is incredibly

[53] Adams, Mike. "Merck vaccine scientist Dr. Maurice Hilleman admitted presence of SV40, AIDS and cancer viruses in vaccines." Natural News. Sept. 15, 2011. Retrieved from http://www.naturalnews.com/033584_Dr_Maurice_Hilleman_SV40.html.
[54] N.A. "Immunization schedules." Centers for Disease Control. Jan. 31, 2014. Retrieved from http://www.cdc.gov/vaccines/schedules/.
[55] Goldman, G. S., and N. Z. Miller. "Relative trends in hospitalizations and mortality among infants by the number of vaccine doses and age, based on the Vaccine Adverse Event Reporting System (VAERS), 1990–2010." Human & Experimental Toxicology 31, no. 10 (2012): 1012-1021.

low, yet all children receive two doses in their first year of life. Not only is hepatitis B rarely fatal, but breastfeeding has also been shown to effectively protect infants from developing chronic infections.[56]

The scientific community has conducted large studies in Finland, Denmark, and the United States examining the association of vaccinations with specific side effects and secondary health disorders. Currently these studies have been reported to show no increase in serious risks or side effects among vaccination recipients.[57] However, these findings contradict other large participant studies. In Australia and New Zealand, an ongoing research study, now including over thirteen thousand participants, continually examines the health status of unvaccinated children in comparison to known statistics for vaccinated kids. The findings have been remarkable. Significantly reduced prevalence of asthma, hay fever, neuro-dermatitis, sinusitis, and otitis media have been seen in the unvaccinated group, typically having less than half the prevalence of these disorders compared to vaccinated children.[58] Likewise rates of attention deficit hyperactivity disorder, epilepsy, migraines, and diabetes mellitus were also substantially less for the unvaccinated group.[59] These objective statistics in addition to numerous subjective reports by parents indicating concern about the health risks of vaccines should highlight the importance of pursuing greater knowledge in this area. Yet large organizations such as the CDC and NIH have failed to pursue such studies.

---

[56] Kenny, Tim. "Breastfeeding." *Patient.co.uk*. July 7, 2013. Retrieved from http://www.patient.co.uk/health/breast-feeding.

[57] American Academy of Pediatrics. "Vaccine safety: Examine the evidence." *AAP. Org*. April 2013. Retrieved from http://www2.aap.org/immunization/families/faq/vaccinestudies.pdf.

[58] VaccineInjury.info. "State of health of unvaccinated children." N.D. Retrieved from http://www.vaccineinjury.info/results-unvaccinated/results-illnesses.html.

[59] Ibid.

The New Zealand study also demonstrated autism to be significantly less among unvaccinated children in comparison to known prevalence rates. In their survey, less than 0.5 percent of unvaccinated children were affected by autism, while average prevalence rates among the vaccinated population exceeds 1.1 percent.[60] This information adds important insights into causation of autism especially as the incidence of the disorder continues to rise dramatically. In 2014, the CDC reported a 30-percent increase in autism over the last two years, representing a thirtyfold increase since the 1960s. Today one in every sixty-eight children is affected by autism, while one in every forty-two boys is affected.[61] Conventional medicine still has no clear idea about causation, but numerous agencies suspect toxins, pesticides, and/or lead as primary suspects. Likewise heavy metals and other components of vaccines are similarly suspected by numerous organizations.

The ability to identify the cause of autism and other childhood disorders is challenging. In part cumulative effects of multiple vaccines and their ingredients affect individuals differently and are difficult to quantify, but even so research pursuing these answers is rarely done. Likewise detecting contaminants within vaccinations and understanding how vaccines interact with our immune systems remain areas where research is lacking. Studies like those conducted in New Zealand provide ongoing cumulative data that demonstrates unvaccinated children clearly have better health outcomes in comparison to vaccinated populations. Therefore the question must be asked as to why the majority of developed nations not only insist on childhood

---

[60] Ibid.

[61] Jaslow, Ryan. "Autism rates rise 30 percent in two-year span: CDC." *CBS News*, 2014. Retrieved from http://www.cbsnews.com/news/autism-rates-rise-30-percent-in-two-year-span-cdc/.

vaccination administration but continually increase the number of vaccines required.

In medical school I was instructed to first do no harm. This was the basic mantra before instituting any treatment, procedure, or diagnostic test. But when it comes to vaccinations, this rule of healthcare seems to be conveniently ignored. Without a doubt some vaccinations have provided clear benefits in advancing health. However, the number of vaccines administered today and the mandatory insistence of their administration on children in public school goes beyond what seems reasonable. For one, vaccines contain toxins and undetectable agents that can affect health in a negative way; secondly, they may interfere with our bodies' own abilities to maintain health over time.

Vaccines as Potential Toxins

The essence of a vaccine is to introduce components of a virus or other infectious agents to a person's immune system, which serves to trigger an immune response. The components usually involve proteins specific to that infectious organism and are known as antigens, or less commonly a small dose of the infectious organism is provided that is too small to cause the actual illness yet enough to stimulate an immune response. After the vaccine is administered and the immune system has had adequate time to develop a response, that person is protected from succumbing to the actual illness later if exposed to the infection. Due to the vaccine, the immune system is now prepared to attack the infection quickly and sufficiently. Thus while the viral particles or protein antigens could represent toxic substances to our health, vaccines use either tiny amounts or noninfectious particles to accomplish their goals without exposing us to infectious quantities.

This rationale for vaccines seems logical. However, in reality a few problems exist. Vaccines by themselves are unable to be stored long term without additional substances to help provide stability and durability. Likewise some vaccines can become infected or contaminated with other infectious organisms, thus requiring additional measures (and additives) to safeguard against these secondary problems. The adjunctive components of vaccinations likely have significant implications on human health. History has shown this to be true and has also shown that some contaminants in vaccines have gone unrecognized, causing many vaccine recipients to be subjected to new infectious organisms.[62] While the vaccine was developed to prevent one infection, it can serve to transmit another or cause toxic effects to our health. These are notable areas of risk, and the benefit received by many vaccines seems insufficient to justify these risks.

One preservative receiving a great deal of attention is thimerosal. Thimerosal contains organic mercury and serves to prolong the shelf life of vaccines, enhance chemical stability, and provide some degree of antiseptic properties. For decades thimerosal has been used in vaccines and continues to be present in many vaccinations worldwide, but concerns over mercury toxicity remain.[63] In fact organic mercury is known to be highly toxic to our health. Specifically, mercury is known to affect the central nervous system and neurodevelopment, and symptoms affecting intellect, memory, personality, and sleep abilities are most common. Research has been conducted failing to link thimerosal to autism or other problems in children, but, despite

[62] Moritz, 2011.

[63] Prate, Dawn. "The great thimerosal cover-up: Mercury, vaccines, autism and your child's health." *Natural News*. Sept. 22, 2005. Retrieved from http://www.naturalnews.com/011764_thimerosal_mercury.html.

this, thimerosal has been banned in the United States for single-dose vial vaccines. This and the fact that international agencies are similarly considering thimerosal's restriction of use should cause some concern.[64]

Unfortunately I have had personal experience with mercury poisoning and related side effects. After years of suffering from poor memory, reduced concentration, personality changes, and anxiety, I eventually underwent a comprehensive toxin screening. As it turned out, the mercury levels in my body were significantly elevated, indicating chronic exposure. While I might have been exposed to organic mercury through eating fish or through dental amalgams that were approximately 50-percent mercury, the most likely source of my exposure was repeated allergy vaccinations. Between first and tenth grades, I regularly received allergy shots that contained thimerosal, and the accumulation of organic mercury in my body over this time presumably resulted in my elevated levels. Mercury alone might not have been enough to account for my complaints later, but the toxic effects to my nervous system throughout the years likely predisposed me to further health injuries from other chemical substances and exposures.

Other toxic preservatives are also used commonly within vaccines. For example, aluminum salts are often included within vaccines to enhance the immunologic response of the vaccine. Others additives include formaldehyde, which serves to kill bacterial and viral contaminants, and monosodium glutamate (MSG), which provides vaccine stability. Each of these agents is foreign to our bodies, and they have the potential to trigger chronic inflammatory reactions

---

[64] Ibid.

within our nervous systems.[65] In turn this chronic inflammatory response can affect a variety of neurological functions, including our ability to remember, our attention and concentration, our moods, and our intellect.

Aluminum can additional contribute to fatigue and muscles weakness and may weaken bone structures. Formaldehyde can result in chronic headaches, fatigue, and insomnia. And MSG can trigger a variety of symptoms such as nausea, facial tingling, headaches, and weakness.[66] The amount of these additives in vaccinations may not seem like much in terms of quantity, but when we appreciate that these agents are being administered to infants weighing less than twenty pounds, the amount can be seen from a different perspective. In addition, no one has a good understanding of how these additives affect health when given in combination. Many researchers assume the effects are additive when in fact they may well be exponential.

So far we have only talked about the potential toxins present in vaccines that are known. What about those that are unknown? In the late 1950s Merck was involved in developing an array of vaccines. In addition to the Sabin polio vaccine, which was an oral vaccine containing live poliovirus, researchers were also working on vaccinations as well as viral studies in general. Maurice Hilleman, the renowned vaccine researcher and developer, worked for Merck, and he discovered that one of the obscure viruses he was studying had contaminated Sabin's polio vaccine. The virus known as SV40, which originated from a species of chimpanzees, was suspected of causing a

---

[65] Adams, Mike. "What's really in vaccines? Proof of MSG, formaldehyde, aluminum and mercury." *Natural News*. October 24, 2012. Retrieved from http://www.natural-news.com/037653_vaccine_additives_thimerosal_formaldehyde.html.
[66] Ibid.

variety of cancers in other species, including humans. Brain tumors, lymphomas, and sarcomas were among the potential concerns. And despite over forty different viruses being inactivated within the vaccine already with formaldehyde, this SV40 virus persisted within the vaccine.[67] The problem was not only resistance to formaldehyde but also the fact that this virus was previously unknown to researchers.

The same concern surrounds the origin of the AIDS virus known as HIV (human immunodeficiency virus). Throughout the 1970s genetic engineering and viral mixing were part of cutting-edge research within the scientific community. President Nixon had declared a war on cancer, and a special virus cancer program was developed at the NCI. Interestingly, the US Army's biological warfare unit located at Fort Detrick was brought under the NCI during this time period. As part of the NCI's discoveries, the enzyme reverse transcriptase was discovered, and experiments using retroviruses in cancers were explored in terms of effects.[68] This constellation of events seems oddly coincidental considering AIDS was first discovered in 1978. Could HIV perhaps been created through manmade research and transmitted through some type of contamination event?

The answer to this question seems to be very likely given some additional pieces of information. In 1978 a group of 1,083 homosexual men was recruited from Manhattan to receive the hepatitis B vaccine, which had been developed by Merck and the National Institute of Health (NIH).[69] Concern over the health of gay men, particularly in relation to sexually transmitted diseases such as hepatitis B, en-

[67] Adams, 2011.

[68] Horowitz, Leonard G. *Emerging Viruses: AIDS, Ebola & Vaccinations.* Tetrahedron, 1997.

[69] Cantwell, Alan. "The gay experiment that started AIDS in America." Rense.com. Nov. 27, 2005. Retrieved from http://www.rense.com/general68/gayex.htm.

couraged research as well as vaccination programs. Therefore these select group of men were chosen for a late-phase trial of the vaccine.[70] While the vaccine proved to be effective, with 96 percent of recipients developing antibodies against the hepatitis B virus, approximately 20 percent of these same men were found to be HIV positive in 1980, making them the largest group of individuals infected with this new virus. While other theories support the onset of HIV occurring as a result of man becoming infected by a chimpanzee virus, these figures involving gay men in Manhattan are significantly higher than the rates of HIV infection at the same time in Africa, where the supposed "species jump" occurred.[71]

The figures above suggest HIV was less likely a "natural" evolution of a virus's ability to move into a new host and more likely something introduced through scientific, manmade technologies. The hepatitis-B vaccination first became available in 1983 while I was attending the University of Alabama in Tuscaloosa as a medical student. Because healthcare workers were identified as being at higher risk for contracting hepatitis B from infected patients, the vaccination was recommended to all medical students. Naturally trusting in our conventional healthcare system, I complied and eventually received three series of vaccinations over several months. But I later learned that potential adverse effects were common with this vaccine similar to other vaccinations due to other chemical agents in the formulation. Mercury, aluminum, and other chemicals present in vaccines have been linked to many side effects, and the chronic inflammatory response triggered by the vaccine itself can cause numerous complaints. Among the most common complaints about the hepatitis-B vaccine

[70] Ibid.
[71] Ibid.

are fatigue, inability to concentrate, blackouts, seizures, depression, insomnia, apathy, and anxiety. Of course medical experts will be the first to point out that such symptoms are nonspecific in nature and could be attributed to many causes. But exactly how many individuals must have these side effects before a causal link is accepted?

Hepatitis-B vaccination protocols are initiated immediately at birth for most infants today. The early administration has been justified as being necessary in order to prevent maternal-to-infant transmission of the virus and to offer the best means to eliminate the hepatitis B virus in infants.[72] But while the risk of hepatitis B may be reduced in children from such practices, some children are also being adversely affected by vaccine components or by the chronic inflammation triggered by the vaccine. By the time infants reach six months of age in the United States, they have already received vaccination exposure to sixty-nine antigens. And these antigens are being given to immature immune systems that remain poorly understood by the conventional medical community.[73] Between allergy shots and subsequent vaccinations received, I have little doubt my complaints were intimately related to these events. How much more would I have been affected had I received these immunizations even earlier in life?

Vaccines have been touted as being a significant advancement of modern medical science, and indeed some global epidemics have been effectively reduced or eradicated through vaccination programs. But the onslaught of vaccinations that are recommended or even required

---

[72] Vara, Christine. "Why Hepatitis B vaccine is not a lifestyle vaccine." *Shot of Prevention*, 2012. Retrieved from http://shotofprevention.com/2012/02/27/why-hepatitis-b-vaccine-is-not-a-lifestyle-vaccine/.

[73] Gervais, Roger R. "Understanding the vaccine controversy." *Nature Life Magazine*, 1996. Retrieved from http://www.naturallifemagazine.com/naturalparenting/vaccines.htm.

today of children raises serious concerns. If such vaccinations are so beneficial then why have allergy rates increased over the last few decades among children? If vaccinations are so effective, why have infant mortality rates increased in countries like the United States? And why have conditions like autism, chronic fatigue syndrome, and fibromyalgia become more prevalent without explanation?[74] Ample evidence suggests that vaccinations may not only be unnecessary in many cases but may also expose individuals to toxins and harmful substances and trigger negative physiologic reactions.

Alternative Motives and Alternative Options

Unfortunately vaccination programs have not always been utilized for healthcare promotion. In 2011 *The Washington Post* wrote an article exposing the Central Intelligence Agency (CIA) in its use of a hepatitis-B vaccination program in Afghanistan as a front to collect DNA material from individuals. The purpose of this collection was to help identify the whereabouts of Osama bin Laden.[75] Such practices have created a great deal of mistrust among some countries regarding vaccination programs, and these concerns are beginning to spread. Not only are motives of espionage and surveillance being increasingly suspected from vaccination programs abroad, but in addition motives such as capitalistic advantage and population control efforts are being considered by many groups.

The obvious alternative motive for vaccination programs outside

---

[74] Ibid.

[75] Ukman, Jason. "CIA defends running vaccine program to find bin Laden." *The Washington Post*, 2011. Retrieved from http://www.washingtonpost.com/world/national-security/cia-defends-running-vaccine-program-to-find-bin-laden/2011/07/13/gIQAbLcFDI_story.html.

of healthcare objectives involves financial gain. Since the development of vaccination mandates in the 1950s and 1960s, many pharmaceutical companies have recognized the potential for profits and financial gain from these therapies. Over the last four decades the number of vaccinations recommended by the CDC has grown exponentially, but despite this increase in vaccinations, the actual improvement in health among children and adolescents can be attributed to better sanitation and clean drinking water. And the number of children with asthma, diabetes, learning disabilities, and attention deficit disorder has increased.[76] As of 2006 the vaccination industry generated a whopping $4.3 billion in revenues in the United States and among five European nations alone. By the year 2016 this figure is expected to increase to $16 billion by some estimates.[77] This statistic is further supported by the fact that approximately 145 additional vaccines are currently in the pipeline for federal approval, ranging from vaccines against meningitis and pneumonia to additional booster vaccines throughout the life spectrum. And if this is not convincing enough, consider the $19 million a day spent by pharmaceutical companies on lobbyist expenses.[78] By following the money trail, and by appreciating how overall health has not significantly improved (and in fact has declined by many accounts), it becomes evident that motivations other than health benefits drive vaccine development.

More recent concerns regarding vaccines involve their use to control global population. According to health theories, the ability to vaccinate impoverished populations throughout the world and

---

[76] Mercola, Joseph. "Blood on Their Hands: The World's Slickest Con Job and a Stack of Deadly LIES..." *Mercola.Com*, 2010. Retrieved from http://articles.mercola.com/sites/articles/archive/2010/11/04/big-profits-linked-to-vaccine-mandates.aspx.
[77] Ibid.
[78] Ibid.

to simultaneously raise their standards of healthcare and education encourages better population control. In countries where educational levels are highest and where development is advanced, population growth approaches zero.[79] Reproductive health and education are additional aspects of such theories. As a result vaccinations are included in this paradigm; however, exactly how vaccines control population growth is somewhat unclear. Do vaccinations prolong life among the impoverished, allowing them to gain a better education, eventually resulting in population control? This seems like a bit of a stretch. Or do vaccines in some other way affect human health so that population growth is curbed?

Bill Gates has been widely recognized as being a proponent of vaccines particularly among impoverished regions of the world, and he likewise is an advocate of depopulation due to CO_2 accumulation issues and global environmental changes.[80] As he is an individual with a vision of the larger picture, could it be that vaccines are a vessel by which population reduction is being methodically planned? As noted previously, the CIA has certainly used vaccination programs for alternative motives.[81] Would it be so farfetched for powerful political actors on the international stage to utilize this tactic as well to achieve their own missions and objectives?

Other motivations for an ever-expanding vaccination schedule also consider the need to continuously fuel a massive healthcare industry. The nature of capitalism is of course growth and progress, and without increasing markets, market shares, and profits, capitalism

[79] Lutz, Wolfgang, and K. C. Samir. "Global human capital: Integrating education and population." *Science* 333, 6042 (2011): 587-592.
[80] Gates, Bill. "Innovating to zero." TED, 2010. Retrieved from http://www.ted.com/talks/bill_gates/transcript.
[81] Ukman, 2011.

stagnates and systems decline. As noted, vaccines over the course of time have been found to contain toxins and contaminants that are detrimental to health. These health disorders subsequently demand evaluations, diagnostics, and treatments, all of which benefit the financial aspects of the healthcare industry. At the same time we have seen how viral contaminations of vaccines have occurred, potentially resulting in the spread of infectious organisms or the development of new infectious diseases. Similarly these occurrences have demanded healthcare services. AIDS alone essentially created an entirely new branch of healthcare services not previously in place.

The definitive evidence regarding these alternative motivations remains unproven; however, support for these ideas is equally as strong as the evidence that vaccines are safe and should be received by every individual. In the United States, where individuals should have the right to determine for themselves whether or not a healthcare treatment is beneficial for them, a push for vaccination mandates is being increasingly experienced. Likewise the vilification of those choosing not to vaccinate their children by groups within the healthcare industry seems to be more pronounced. These developments combined with the many questions about the benefits and risks of vaccines raise great suspicion about the real motivation for vaccination programs today.

Ultimately the question must be asked whether or not vaccines are absolutely necessary. By many accounts the actual morbidity and mortality for diseases for which vaccines are administered are relatively low. The risk, therefore, for choosing not to vaccinate a child or oneself also appears to be quite small. For example, some of the most common of these disorders for which vaccinations are received involve pertussis or whooping cough, which averages ten thousand cases per year in the United States but is rarely fatal. Likewise chickenpox averages fifty thousand cases per year and similarly has low mortality rates.[82] Based on the information available, recommending vaccinations for children cannot be done without serious considerations and concern. Instead of the plethora of vaccinations currently received by most children, a limited number of vaccines should be administered. These would be only those that protect children from high-risk health disorders based on incidence, prevalence, and endemic factors. By my assessment, no vaccinations would be recommended for many children, while maybe up to two would be recommended for others. The better approach is to take a more natural strategy toward boosting the immune system while avoiding the potential risks of vaccines altogether.[83]

In these latter cases parents are choosing options like breastfeeding infants for up to twelve months of age; providing supplemental dosages of vitamins A, D3, and C; including ample fresh fruits and vegetables in the diet; providing other supplements such as glutathione, curcumin, zinc, flavonoids, and ginger; and ensuring adequate sleep schedules. These measures in addition to avoiding toxins, preservatives, and concentrated sugars boost a person's immune system while avoiding potential substances, like vaccinations, that may weaken it.[84] Despite what conventional medicine suggests, beneficial alternatives to vaccines do exist. Considering these options is important for optimal immune health, and by selecting these options instead

---

[82] Mercola, 2010.

[83] Sears, Robert W. *The vaccine book: Making the right decision for your child*. Hachette Digital, Inc., 2011.

[84] Neustaedter, Randall. "What are the alternatives to vaccinations?" *HealthyChild.com*. Retrieved from http://www.healthychild.com/what-are-the-alternatives-to-vaccination/.

of vaccines, the risks that appear evident from vaccine formulations are avoided completely.

In summary, the information circulating in the mainstream media and through conventional medical channels regarding vaccines appears on the surface to be convincing of their benefits and safety profiles. But these reports fail to tell the complete picture. The history of vaccine development and growth of this field over the last century is far from straightforward, and several concerns exist in relation to their overall effects and safety. From contaminants to toxic components, evidence suggests vaccines have contributed to the development of many illnesses and health disorders. And despite drops in infectious disease numbers, overall health and infant mortality rates have not improved over this course of time. This information, combined with statistics and accounts that relate the use of vaccines for alternative motives other than health, poses additional concerns. With this information, however, and an awareness that alternatives to vaccines do exist, choices can be made by parents and individuals alike. In doing so, the right to choose which healthcare treatment is best is preserved.

CHAPTER 5

Dietary Factors: You Are What You Eat

My father is approaching ninety-seven years of age and is incredibly healthy. In addition to living through the Great Depression, serving the nation in World War II, and being the son of a Pennsylvania coal miner, my father has lived an extensive life as a world-class musician with exceptional talents involving the flute, cello, and bass. Without question his life has been a series of challenges, but consistently he has emphasized diet as an important aspect of health. His dedication to natural and organic foods as well as attention to necessary vitamins and supplements has played a significant role in his continued health and longevity. However, increasingly today many of us have fewer and fewer opportunities to make such important dietary choices. Everywhere around us are invisible and unknown ingredients in food-stuffs, and even foods that appear to be natural may contain geneti-cally modified components or contaminants. As a result most people do not even realize their poor decisions regarding food even when the best intentions are present.

Food is energy for our bodies and minds. The better the source of food we eat, the more likely we will enjoy good health. But exactly what represents good food in the twenty-first century? Grocery stores contain plenty of fresh fruit and vegetables, which should be ideal for our diets. However, many of these foods have been exposed to chemicals, pesticides, and insecticides that persist in residual amounts and threaten our health. Likewise scientific efforts to create foods with natural resistance to pests and insects have allowed increased food production, but the effects of these efforts on the nutritional value and on our own health have been poorly explored. Even the water we drink is no longer assured of being free of such toxins. In this chapter we will explore all of these concerns regarding our diets in addition to many other substances that are commonly found in foodstuffs today. By having a better awareness of these issues and better choices about what we eat, better decisions about our health can subsequently be made.

Genetically Modified Foods

Many people may have heard of GMO foods, but few likely understand exactly what "GMO" means or the effects such foods have on our health. GMO stands for "genetically modified organisms," and increasingly these foods have become a routine part of most Americans' diets. In essence, GMO development occurred as a means to reduce the amount of pesticide use agriculturally while increasing the productivity of farms and crop producers. While this sounds like admirable goals, the reality of GMO foods may in the long run be counterproductive to these objectives. As is the case with many new technologies that are poorly researched, the risks and adverse events related to the advancement may not be known until many years later.

The process of genetic modification involves identifying a sequence of DNA that offers some advantage to a plant or crop. For example, a DNA sequence may offer resistance to certain pests or disease. Once such a genetic sequence is identified, scientists place the sequence into the DNA of a bacterium and then "infect" a plant with this organism. Once the plant is infected, scientists then treat it with antibiotics, which kills all the plant cells that failed to incorporate the new genetically modified bacterium, leaving only the new GMO cells. This new breed of plant is then cloned and reproduced for the agricultural industry.[85] In theory the new plant is now resistant to insects and pests common to that crop, allowing reduced amounts of pesticides to be used. Likewise GMO may also infer enhanced productivity to the plant, resulting in higher crop yields.[86]

Unfortunately evidence now supports that these "benefits" do not reflect reality and that unexpected side effects are being identified. While the DNA insertions are supposed to result in single effects, it is now evident that such a change in DNA structure has multiple effects on organism activity. As a result some unsuspected genes are activated, causing an array of unknown effects.[87] And with activation of these additional genes, the nutritional value of plants declines since energy is being spent on other metabolic processes. In addition, over time the effects of insect and pest resistance conferred by the GMO process declines as pests and insects adapt through natural selection and evolution. Ultimately this results in an increase (rather than a

---

[85] Natural Revolution. "The good, bad and ugly about GMOs." *NaturalRevolution.Org*, 2013. Retrieved from http://naturalrevolution.org/gmo-resources/the-good-bad-and-ugly-about-gmos/.

[86] Ibid.

[87] GMO Awareness. "GMO risks." *GM-Awareness.Com*, 2011. Retrieved from http://gmo-awareness.com/all-about-gmos/gmo-risks/.

decrease) of pesticide and insecticide use, and the agents subsequently required may actually be more potent than traditional agents.[88]

Other harmful effects from GMO foods involve the propagation of these genetic modifications throughout the biosphere. Changes in the DNA structure within GMO foods have been found to incorporate themselves into intestinal bacteria of the gut. This means DNA alterations can be identified in other organisms or cells, resulting in a variety of unknown effects.[89] Also the genetic changes in plants cause other organisms to be affected within the environment. For example, the Monarch butterfly as well as certain bee populations have declined presumably due to changes in various GMO crops. The result of these changes thus causes not only potential detrimental effects to human health but also widespread biologic pollution throughout the environment.[90] While GMO foods may have been started with good intentions, the long-term effects seem to be counterproductive to their objectives.

A major problem with GMO foods involves the overwhelming lack of scientific investigation into their effects and safety. Recent literature searches demonstrated that only forty-one articles explored GMO food safety, and of these only nineteen involved human study.[91] Likewise large agricultural and chemical corporations have consistently propagated biased research and information positioning GMO foods as favorable. This strategy is accomplished by withholding GMO seeds for study, maintaining control over research publication approval, infiltrating FDA and USDA committees with ex-employees,

---

[88] Ibid.
[89] Ibid.
[90] Ibid.
[91] Natural Revolution, 2013.

and infusing millions of dollars into lobbyist efforts.[92] Their efforts have been successful toward this mission as evidenced by the fact that GMO food labels have still not been required in the United States due to their opposition to such legislation.

In European countries the use of GMO foods has been banned, which further supports evidence that these products are likely detrimental to human as well as environmental health. Only in the United States are GMO foods being developed and manufactured for large-scale use. The FDA has no specific safety requirements for GMO foods in terms of testing, and mandatory labeling is not required as of yet.[93] Despite this, evidence exists that GMO foods can introduce new allergens, expose us to new toxins, and create new diseases as a result of genetic alterations. The only way we can currently avoid such compounds in the United States is to buy purely organic products, which by law cannot contain any GMO components.[94] Only then can we escape the broad influence of GMO foods and the industries supporting their use.

Chemical Food Residues

In earlier chapters the discussion of pesticides and their potentially harmful health effects was explored in detail. While I was exposed to chlordane through probable pesticide in foodstuffs, numerous other pesticides pose similar threats to human health as chemical residues on the foods we routinely eat. In addition numerous other chemicals are administered to plants as well as livestock, which have

---

[92] Ibid.
[93] Ibid.
[94] GMO Awareness, 2011.

the potential to gain access to our bodies and interfere with normal metabolic processes and immune system function. Despite efforts by governmental agencies to ensure our safety in this regard through standards, its ability to provide significant assurances is limited by regulatory procedures and by the complexity of chemical interactions that may occur. This combined with economic incentives to seek favorable results from chemical practices often places health and safety in a backseat.

Let's consider pesticide use again in relation to agricultural production. The US Department of Agriculture (USDA) and the Food and Drug Administration (FDA) have established maximal residual limits (or MRLs) of various pesticides, herbicides, and insecticides that may persist on or in vegetables and fruits sold for our consumption. These "tolerances" reportedly are safe amounts that through safety testing have failed to produce significant disease or illness.[95] As a result most of us assume the foods we then purchase from our grocers are safe, and though we acknowledge that chemicals have been used to produce these foods and may persist in small amounts, these are insufficient to cause health problems.

A few problems with this rationale exist, however. In researching the potential effects of these chemicals, the USDA and FDA both tend to take a simplistic view of each substance. Each chemical is tested in isolation through animal and human experiments to determine MRLs, but rarely do such chemicals get utilized in such ways. More often than not, more than one pesticide, herbicide, insecticide, or chemical agent is used within the agricultural industry, and thus synergistic effects on health of these chemical combinations are not

---

[95] PANNA. "Pesticides on food." *Pesticide Action Network North America*, n.d. Retrieved from http://www.panna.org/issues/food-agriculture/pesticides-on-food.

adequately explored.[96] Secondly, as I noted within my own body, chemicals like chlordane can accumulate and become stored within tissues of the body for decades. Research typically does not examine the accumulation effects of being exposed to various chemicals over time and their effects on health.[97] Thirdly, evaluations involving the exact timing of chemical exposures are rarely assessed. In children particularly, timing of exposure can be a critical variable in terms of health effects since their growth and development are at an accelerated pace.[98] Thus while safety experiments are conducted, the ability of these experiments to mimic reality is limited.

The other major shortcoming of safety evaluations also involves the ability to test the long-term effects of such chemicals on health. Exposure to chemical residuals in food today may not result in significant health effects for twenty years or more. By the time such research would reveal such effects, many newer chemical agents will be on the market. Keeping pace with research and development of these new substances becomes a serious challenge when considering safety evaluations. Unfortunately the FDA and USDA have a policy wherein many compounds are considered harmless until proven harmful. This approach is distinctly different from other countries such as European nations that assume just the opposite.[99]

Admittedly the FDA and USDA acknowledge that long-term reports of the effects of chemical residuals on foods are lacking, but these agencies still produce annual reports concerning MRLs and routine food testing. According to the Environmental Working

---

[96] Ibid.
[97] Ibid.
[98] Ibid.
[99] Ibid.

Group, which examines more than 100,000 of these reports, numerous foods have been found to contain an array of chemical residues. In fact the group cited twelve foods as the "dirty dozen" with each having between forty-seven and sixty-seven different pesticide residuals on them. Such foods included celery, lettuce, apples, strawberries, blueberries, potatoes, grapes, spinach, and more.[100] In addition, even among organic crops, which are supposedly free of such chemicals, approximately 50 percent have routinely tested positive for some chemical residues.[101] These findings demonstrate the need for concern among consumers about food safety and about how such chemicals can be avoided.

Health effects associated with pesticide, insecticide, and herbicide residuals can be numerous as well as somewhat nonspecific. Attention deficit hyperactivity disorder has been linked to chlordane, and other agents are suspected of causing autism spectrum disorders.[102] But while birth defects, neurologic impairments, and cancer risks have been identified with many of these chemicals, other side effects may be less obvious. Fatigue, memory loss, muscle aches, joint aches, poor concentration, and personality changes are just some of the vaguer and more generalized complaints higher doses of these chemicals may cause. I actually experienced these vaguer symptoms during medical school and residency, which was likely in part due to chemical exposure throughout my childhood. Because these complaints are less "tangible" and testable, the ability to associate chemical residues

---

[100] Dellorto, Danielle. "'Dirty Dozen' carries more pesticide residue, group says." *CNN.Com*, 2010. Retrieved from http://www.cnn.com/2010/HEALTH/06/01/dirty.dozen.produce.pesticide/.

[101] Saliba, Andrea. "The poison in our food." *The McGill Daily*, 2014. Retrieved from http://www.mcgilldaily.com/2014/01/the-poison-in-our-food/.

[102] Ibid.

on foods to these health problems poses serious research challenges. Instead of playing it safe, however, the USDA and FDA choose to roll the dice.

Pesticides and plant chemicals are unfortunately not the only chemical residues we must worry about. The agricultural industry since the middle part of the last century has adopted the use of antibiotics and hormones in livestock as a means to enhance productivity and efficiency as well. Both of these agents have been shown to increase growth and development of livestock, reduce the feed requirements, and enhance production of byproducts like milk.[103] Since the 1950s an array of different antibiotics has been used to treat swine, cattle, and poultry by adding this to their feed. Over time several of these antibiotic agents have been banned due to the development of antibiotic-resistant bacteria that posed health threats to humans. Not only can antibiotic administration result in more aggressive strains of bacteria that can affect human health, but these same antibiotics reach the soil through livestock excrement, affecting plants, other animals, and our water supply (through soil runoff).[104] But like with pesticide chemicals, the FDA and USDA always seem to be behind the curve. Only after a specific antibiotic is found to cause a new strain of bacteria that threatens health is action taken to ban the use of the antibiotic. Rarely are proactive measures taken.

Similarly the use of hormones like estrogen and progesterone in livestock has progressively increased over the last several decades. In fact diethylstilbestrol (DES), which is known to cause vaginal

---

[103] Natural Standard. "Hormones and antibiotics in food supply." Health24.Com, 2011. Retrieved from http://www.health24.com/Lifestyle/Environmental-health/21st-century-life/Hormones-and-antibiotics-in-food-supply-20130311.
[104] Ibid.

cancer in women, was used in poultry and cattle commonly before 1970 to enhance growth.[105] While DES is no longer approved, the use of hormonal steroids in livestock remains FDA approved, including the use of bovine growth hormone or BGH. Many agricultural farms no longer use BGH because of potential health effects related to cancer and premature sexual development in children, but still an estimated 30 percent of farms in the United States administer BGH to their cattle for milk production. This continues despite BGH being banned in Europe, Canada, Japan, Australia, and New Zealand.[106]

In appreciating these developments and the nature of health risks placed on individuals from these various chemicals, one must ask why a more cautious approach is not employed. According to the USDA, approximately 45 percent of crops would spoil without the application of pesticides.[107] Certainly the ability to produce more food products from crops and livestock that require fewer costs is attractive to many producers throughout the industry. Thus the standard answer as to why such chemical residues are allowed is based on the assumption that demand warrants such measures. Without these chemicals inadequate food supplies would be experienced, driving up prices and limiting access to basic food needs.[108] But one must question whether this accurately portrays the entire picture.

Before Monsanto sold its BGH division to Eli Lilly, the revenues generated annually from BGH sales to the farming industry totaled over $270 million.[109] This amount of revenue certainly gets one's

---

[105] Ibid.
[106] Ibid.
[107] Dellorto, 2010.
[108] Natural Standard, 2011.
[109] Ibid.

attention and highlights the important relationship between the agricultural and chemical industries. If only a minority of farmers are providing BGH to their livestock, and this degree of income results then imagine the revenues resulting from all pesticides, insecticides, antibiotics and more. Indeed these chemicals have allowed greater efficiencies and productivities in getting foodstuffs to the market and onto consumers' dinner tables, but at the same time they also generate billions of dollars for corporations. With an organic food industry gaining momentum and size, the belief that the use of these chemicals in meeting consumer demand is a necessary evil becomes less and less acceptable. Taking a fresh look at the foods we eat and the chemicals used to produce them is required if we want to truly attend to our long-term health and wellbeing.

Water Contaminants—The Invisible Threats

Unlike with many foodstuffs, many people today purposefully choose to drink bottled water or employ some type of filtration system to purify their drinking water at home. These practices may be a result of convenience or due to a preferred taste, but they likewise may result from some awareness that contaminants in our standard drinking water are common. Over the last several decades, water treatment facilities and water utility companies have made efforts to purify water according to Environmental Protection Agency (EPA) standards, but despite these efforts unscreened contaminants still exist. In an anonymous study involving twenty-five such utility centers, water samples were tested for contamination for over 251 chemicals, bacteria, viruses, and microbes. While none of the centers had 117 of these agents, more than two-thirds had twenty-five of these contaminants and about a third had 113 of them.[110]

In the above study the amounts of the contaminants found were low in quantity, but most concerning was that some of the substances found were not routinely regulated by the EPA or by state water and health divisions. For example, the metal strontium was found in samples as was a herbicide named metachlor and various perfluorinated compounds. Metachlor has been labeled a carcinogen, while perfluorinated like PFOS and PFOA have been associated with several poor health conditions. PFOS has been linked to ADHD and thyroid disease, while PFOS has been associated with high cholesterol levels, ulcerative colitis, testicular cancer, and renal cancer.[111] Interestingly, perfluorinated compounds, which are byproducts of the industrial processing of food packaging, fabrics, and cookware, have been found in the bloodstream of almost everyone in the country.[112] Presumably this exposure has been a result in part due to contaminated drinking water.

Just as the FDA and USDA have MRLs for chemical residues, the EPA has maximum contaminant levels (MCLs) for various contaminants. And also like the food industry, the water regulatory agencies lack sufficient information and research concerning long-term health and safety data from cumulative exposure to these small amounts of contaminants over time. Take into consideration for a moment the half-life of some perfluorinated compounds. PFOA has a half-life of four years. In other words half of the amount to which an individual

[110] Bienkowski, Brian. "New report: Unregulated contaminants common in drinking water." *Environmental Health News,* 2013. Retrieved from http://www.environmentalhealthnews.org/ehs/news/2013/unregulated-water-contaminants.

[111] Ibid.

[112] Ibid.

is exposed takes four years to be metabolized. Generally it takes five half-lives for a substance to be completely eliminated, or in the case of PFOA, complete elimination takes twenty years. For PFOS, its half-life is twice as long at eight years, resulting in complete elimination in forty years.[113] It's no wonder these agents can trigger carcinogenic reactions in the body since even small amounts of exposure have the potential to persist for decades.

Industrial byproducts in the drinking water are not the only concern today. Numerous studies over the past decade have also revealed pharmaceutical toxins as being prevalent in the drinking water. Currently more than 50 percent of Americans take at least one prescribed medication, and 10 percent of the population takes an antidepressant medication.[114] Therefore it is not surprising that these agents and metabolic byproducts are showing up in our drinking water as we flush unused prescriptions down the toilet and excrete large amounts of unmetabolized drugs. While research studies as well as media publicity about this subject have been scant, environmental studies in the United States have shown that 80 percent of the rivers and streams sampled test positive for low levels of pharmaceuticals.[115] In 2004 Britain found tap water contained a nearly continuously low level of Prozac® in its content. And in 2008 the EPA found approximately 50 pharmaceutical drugs to exist within the drinking water of 41 million Americans.[116] Just imagine the effects these substances may be having on our health and our children's wellbeing.

---

[113] Safer Chemicals. "Perfluorinated compounds." *SaferChemical.Org.* Retrieved from http://www.saferchemicals.org/resources/chemicals/pfc.html.

[114] Harvey, Matt. "No, you can't drink…water." The Fix, 2013. Retrieved from http://www.thefix.com/content/water-supply-contamination-trace-pharmaceuticals8666.

[115] Ibid.

[116] Ibid.

The problem with pharmaceutical contamination of the water involves the inability of the EPA and water treatment centers to screen, detect, and filter such agents in the purification process. Drugs such as antidepressants, anticonvulsants, and sedatives are commonly found in public water in low levels as a result. The long-term effects of these substances are unknown in relation to human health, and additional harm to the environment and other ecosystems is likely as well. In fact studies examining the effects of sedatives on marine life have demonstrated changes in feeding and migration habits, which could have far-reaching implications on the species. In addition since pharmaceutical contaminants reach natural environmental watersheds, even bottled water has been found to be affected by these contaminants.[117] It seems the effect of conventional medicines on the population and even the environment is broader than pharmaceutical industries may have ever suspected.

While many contaminants in water remain unknown, one of the most significant toxic ingredients in water is a substance with which we are all familiar. Since the late 1940s drinking water in most American cities has been fluoridated under the assumption this chemical provides healthy teeth and reduces cavities. However, the evidence for this effect is rather scant, and even more importantly toxic health effects from fluoride are strongly suspected.[118] The process leading to widespread fluoridation of public water supplies began in the 1930s, when American conglomerates and corporate leaders began to identify ways in which industrial wastes involving sodium fluoride could be reutilized for profit and gain. ALCOA, an aluminum manufac-

---

[117] Ibid.

[118] Information Liberation. "The fluoride conspiracy." 2006. Retrieved from http://www.informationliberation.com/?id=14949.

turer, was the largest producer of fluoride waste at the time, and they teamed up with other companies including DuPont, Colgate, and Kellogg in developing alternative uses for fluoride. Alternative uses not only offered another revenue stream for these corporations but likewise provided solutions for health-related lawsuits involving fluoride toxicity that had been filed against these companies.[119]

To further this venture ALCOA produced laboratory rat studies that demonstrated how fluoride reduced dental cavities, and based on these findings the company pushed for widespread water fluoridation.[120] Despite evidence of fluoride's toxic effects on health (which were likely suppressed or not reviewed), fluoridation policies gained favor as dental and traditional medical professions began to support the idea. Even today tremendous gaps exist in the research supporting fluoride as a truly beneficial agent to dental health. In fact several professional organizations have stated quite the opposite. The International Academy of Oral Medicine and Toxicology has classified fluoride as unapproved due to high toxicity, while the US National Cancer Institute's Toxicological Program has found fluoride to be an equivocal carcinogen.[121] It would seem corporate greed developed a means by which waste byproducts could be turned into profits while ignoring human health interests in the process.

The limited studies that have examined fluoride and its relation to health have suggested significant neurologic effects. Studies out of Harvard in the 1990s demonstrated that fluoride administration to laboratory animals resulted in lower intelligence and higher rates of

---

[119] Ibid.
[120] Ibid.
[121] Ibid.

attention deficit disorder behaviors.[122] Likewise other reports dating back forty years from Kettering suggested toxic effects of fluoride on the lungs and lymph nodes in laboratory rats.[123] Current evidence also supports fluoride as increasing cancer rates, osteoporosis, and dental problems.[124] But despite this evidence millions of people throughout the world continue to drink fluoridated water on a daily basis, failing to realize the potential harm it may bring.

Our bodies are composed of approximately 60 percent water, which is depleted constantly through normal processes of metabolism. Therefore, replenishing water on a daily basis in adequate quantities is a necessity, but at the same time we must be conscious of what other toxins, contaminants, or additives might be included. Options do exist to ensure one's tap water is free of such contaminants and toxins. Private laboratory testing of one's home water sample is a good start after which the choice to invest in a home purification system may be made. Alternatively, distilled water, which has been converted to steam and then cooled back to water, does eliminate the hidden contaminants discussed in this section. Being safe is better than being sorry when evidence eventually surfaces supporting the negative health effects of these various water contaminants.

Harmful Food Ingredients

Thus far foods have been considered from the perspective of their production, manufacturing, and preparation, but additionally ingredients are often added to foods that can be harmful to health as

[122] Ibid.
[123] Ibid.
[124] Ibid.

well. Increasingly, foods are processed to include preservatives, taste enhancers, calorie-reducing agents, and more. And some foods automatically contain substances that, when taken in large quantities, may be toxic to the body. Among some of the most common food ingredients that trigger health concerns are gluten, aspartame, monosodium glutamate (MSG), and nitrite compounds. Each of these has been associated with negative health effects and complaints and therefore deserve specific consideration.

Two prevalent food additives today include aspartame and MSG. Aspartame, which is marketed under brand names like Nutrasweet, Equal, Spoonful, and others, is a sugar substitute offering sweet taste without the calories. MSG on the other hand enhances flavor and taste when combined with more savory foods. Interestingly both aspartame and MSG have something in common other than their influence on taste. Aspartame consists of mostly aspartic acid, while MSG is predominantly glutamic acid. Both of these compounds are excitatory amino acids, which accounts for a great deal of their toxicities.[125] Excitatory amino acids essentially stimulate neurons of the brain and allow a greater influx of calcium into these cells. But the degree of calcium influx encouraged is often toxic to these neurons, causing free radical formation and direct injury. As a result both aspartame and MSG can cause brain cell death when ingested in significant quantities.[126]

As perhaps expected, symptoms that have been reported with both MSG and aspartame have been quite similar. Complaints range

---

[125] Mercola, Joseph. "Aspartame: By far the most dangerous substance added to most foods today." *Mercola.com*, 2011. Retrieved from http://articles.mercola.com/sites/articles/archive/2011/11/06/aspartame-most-dangerous-substance-added-to-food.aspx.
[126] Ibid.

from headaches and migraines to nausea, visual blurring, depression, fatigue, insomnia, memory loss, and joint pain. In addition these substances have been associated with seizures on occasion.[127] Unfortunately despite the fact that more than 75 percent of all adverse events from food additives can be attributed to one of these agents, both aspartame and MSG remain FDA approved.[128] Research supports their negative health effects, but consumption of foods with these excitotoxins are ever-increasing. Ironically the surge in adult and child obesity over the past three decades has encouraged even greater consumption of substances containing aspartame due to its calorie-free nature, but research studies also show that aspartame and diet sodas in general are actually associated with worsening weight gain rather than obesity improvement.[129] The luxury of enhanced food taste seems to be coming at great expense to consumers' health. It continues to be amazing how the FDA allows such substances to persist in our diets yet restricts so many other natural health remedies from routine use.

In addition to aspartic acid, aspartame also contains two other harmful substances that include phenylalanine and methanol. Phenylalanine has been identified as a human toxin, and when large amounts of aspartame-containing drinks and foods are consumed, levels of phenylalanine in the blood have been noted to be elevated. Even in individuals who metabolize phenylalanine normally, the effects of this chemical serves to reduce serotonin levels in the brain.[130] And lower serotonin levels have been associated with major depression

---

[127] Ibid.

[128] Ibid.

[129] Lundy, Karen Saucier, and Sharyn Janes. *Community Health Nursing: Caring for the public's health.* New York, NY: Jones & Bartlett Learning, 2009.

[130] Mercola, 2011.

as well as with memory impairment. Methanol on the other is metabolized to formaldehyde, which has been designated as a cumulative toxin by the EPA. Because methanol is metabolized slowly with a low rate of excretion from the body, small amounts can slowly build to toxic levels over time. Symptoms related to methanol toxicity often involve the visual system, and this substance has also been recognized as a carcinogen and as an agent causing birth defects.[131] Regardless of how great the taste may be, do these food additives sound like something one would want to put into one's body?

Another well-known food additive with known negative health effects is sodium nitrite. This food preservative offers antimicrobial effects while also enhancing the flavor and color of many foods. Most often sodium nitrite is added to processed and cure meats like hot dogs, deli meats, and bacon. But while sodium nitrite preserves and enhances taste, it similarly increases cancer risk. Once in the body sodium nitrite is converted to nitrosamines, and these substances increase the occurrence of several different types of neoplasms. Colon cancer risk is increased by 50 percent with sodium nitrite intake, while bladder cancer, stomach cancer, and pancreatic cancer are increased 59 percent, 38 percent, and 67 percent respectively.[132] According to the World Cancer Research Fund, which reviewed over seven thousand clinical studies involving sodium nitrite, processed meats should be completely avoided.[133]

While aspartame, MSG, and nitrites represent additives that impose harmful health side effects on the body, some food components

---

[131] Ibid.

[132] Mercola, Joseph. "7,000 clinical studies concur—This meat is a clear invitation to cancer..." Mercola.com, 2011. Retrieved from http://articles.mercola.com/sites/articles/archive/2011/04/11/when-are-hotdogs-better-for-you-than-chicken.aspx.

[133] Ibid.

are naturally unhealthy. Foods heavy in saturated fats and sugar content are ones that are easily recognized as unhealthy, but what about ones that are supposedly good for you? For decades now health experts have bombarded the public with messages concerning whole grains, and certainly whole grains have health benefits in terms of lowering cholesterol, reducing colon cancer risk, and promoting good heart function. But at the same time even too much of a good thing can be detrimental. Wheat contains a protein called gluten, which is composed of two main components, gliadins and glutenins. These components are broken down in the small intestines into smaller proteins that are then absorbed, and for the majority of people that is the end of the story.[134] However, for 1 percent of the population these gluten proteins trigger an autoimmune and inflammatory response that causes the body to attack itself, damaging the intestinal wall and other structures throughout the body. These patients are labeled as having celiac disease, and as a result of their condition, they suffer from numerous problems including malnutrition, fatigue, abdominal pain, and digestive difficulties as well as many others. Also notable is that 80 percent of patients with celiac disease at any given time remain undiagnosed.[135]

At first glance a disorder related to wheat affecting only 1 percent of the population may not seem too alarming. But celiac disease only represents the tip of the iceberg. More than 10 percent of the population suffers from a less severe version of the disease labeled "gluten sensitivity." With this condition individuals have the same type of

---

[134] Petersen, Vikki, and Richard Peterson. *The Gluten Effect.* True Health Publishing, 2009.
[135] Ibid.

inflammatory reaction to gluten proteins but to a lesser degree.[136] Regardless, gluten sensitivity has been associated with numerous problems related to autoimmune tissue injury. In addition to the same complaints listed above for celiac disease, patients with gluten sensitivity can develop neuropathy, gait imbalance, diabetes, thyroid disease, multiple sclerosis, fibromyalgia, insomnia, and skin disorders. Gluten sensitivity has even been associated with higher rates of autism, schizophrenia, and some types of epilepsy.[137] Gluten for many people is identified by the body as a foreign invader, and as a result the immune system launches a full-scale attack on it. Unfortunately, however, the attack is not limited to gluten alone, and many other bodily tissues become targets accidentally in the process.

In addition to gluten sensitivity, some evidence now suggests that too many grains are detrimental to brain function in a more general way. Increased occurrence of memory problems, dementia, attention deficit disorders, depression, anxiety, and headaches have been associated with an overload of breads, carbohydrates, and sugars.[138] Likewise rebound cravings for carbohydrates and sugars are well recognized as causing food addictions leading to obesity, diabetes, and other health problems. Moderation and seeking balance in the diet remain important strategies in pursuing dietary health while avoiding the plethora of toxins, poisons, and chemicals. The number of such substances seem to be growing every year. Unfortunately conventional medicine professionals and governmental safety organizations can be unreliable resources in providing proper health guidance when it comes to these concerns.

---

[136] Ibid.

[137] Ibid.

[138] Perlmutter, David. *Grain Brain*. New York, NY: Little, Brown & Co., 2009.

The challenge today involves identifying which foods are safe and which foods are not. Even foods like wheat and whole grains, which are widely promoted by the medical industry, can be damaging to health. Other foods that are genetically modified, foods containing preservatives and additives, and the water we drink (bottled and tap) pose additional risks that are overlooked, ignored, or purposefully allowed to exist due to other nonhealth-related interests. Staying abreast of this information is not only difficult, but it is even more challenging to gain access to objective, nonbiased resources that provide the entire picture. While the scope of this chapter on foods and dietary agents negatively affecting health only scratches the surface, enough information has been shared providing convincing evidence that caution is certainly warranted. Being informed and selective remains the best safeguard for your health, while eating natural, raw, and organic foods offers the best strategy.

CHAPTER 6

Sleep Deprivation: Limiting Health and Healing

Exactly how many hours of sleep does the body need in order to function normally and feel healthy? One might assume the answer to be fairly straightforward, being seven or eight hours, but in reality the range for normal sleep can be as little as four hours a day up to ten hours a day depending on the individual. For those who only need four hours of sleep to function well, they often excel in today's fast-paced world, where time is a critical resource. But for those who require ten hours of sleep daily, they often struggle simply trying to meet basic expectations. In fact these individuals often find they must sacrifice sleep in order to meet their responsibilities, and in the process their health becomes compromised. Even among average sleepers who require eight hours of sleep daily, the temptation to get ahead by sacrificing sleep becomes increasingly powerful.

In the United States polls over the last decade have shown that nearly fifty million individuals are sleep-deprived on a regular basis with nearly two-thirds getting less than seven hours of sleep on average.[139] For a few this may be adequate, but for the majority sleep deprivation has become a chronic reality. While the obvious issues related to sleep deprivation involve levels of alertness and brain function, many other health-related problems are triggered by inadequate sleep. In addition to cognitive setbacks, problems related to the immune system, the hormonal system, and even the cardiovascular system surface when sleep is insufficient. Understanding the role of sleep in relationship to health is thus important in developing positive lifestyle habits. Likewise this knowledge helps avoid societal pressures and temptations to persevere without sleep, knowing such choices are not in the best interest of good health.

Lack of Sleep and Ill Health

Being a medical physician and having trained in residency during the 1980s, I am well experienced with the effects of sleep deprivation on the brain. On a routine basis I would be on call for medical patients for forty-eight consecutive hours at a time, after which patient presentations to faculty and important medical decisions had to be made. The inconsistency between my clinical performance during these rotations and my superior academic scores on national testing becomes understandable when my profound degree of sleep deprivation is considered. Despite an abundance of literature supporting the negative effects of sleep deprivation on cognitive performance and attention even then, medical institutions refused to see the evidence. Like a horse with blinders on lumbering forward down a familiar path, medical professors insisted on maintaining the status quo. Since they had

---

[139] Lawlis, G. Frank. "The Sleep Solution Workbook." DrPhil.com, n.d. Retrieved from http://www.drphil.com/assets/c/c0f3ab7356c5913f1a91dc7c7c347ecc.pdf.

suffered similar residency schedules and had turned out "fine" then a need for change from their perspectives was not necessary.

I recall on several occasions driving off the road or out of my lane while driving home after such long on-call schedules, and periodically throughout the day I would suffer brief periods of micro-sleep when my concentration would completely lapse in the middle of a conversation. Interestingly only after the Institute of Medicine came out with a report in 2008 did residency requirements and schedule mandates appear. The rising incidence of medical errors finally prompted greater attention to chronic sleep deprivation of medical residents, and public and media pressures eventually encouraged change. Subsequently the Accreditation Council for Graduate Medical Education (ACGME) now limits on-call shifts to sixteen hours for first-year medical residents and to twenty-four hours for second-year residents and higher. Likewise medical residents must have at least eight hours off after a routine shift and at least fourteen hours after a twenty-four-hour call session.[140] While these measures are certainly better than call schedules during my tenure in residency, the work demands and limited opportunities to sleep still promote chronic sleep deprivation. But I suppose this is a step in the right direction.

From a neurological perspective sleep is vital to optimal performance of the brain. Every major area of the brain is affected by sleep deprivation. Reduced temporal lobe function has been noted with lack of sleep, causing decreased verbal learning and memory function. Reduced parietal lobe function similarly occurs with reduced abilities to perform mathematics and solve numerical problems. Frontal lobe

---

[140] ACGME. "2010 ACGME Residency Common Program Requirements." *AMA-ASSN.org*, 2010. Retrieved from http://www.ama-assn.org/resources/doc/rfs/dutyhours.pdf.

involvement has been associated with reduced creativity, impaired attention and concentration, and impaired judgment and impulse control. But what has been most revealing as of late is research evidence showing that sleep deprivation causes cell death of brain neurons. In some areas of the brain, as many as 25 percent of neurons can be permanently damaged as a result of chronic sleep deprivation.[141]

With sleep deprivation being so common today, and based on research showing how damaging sleep loss can be to the brain, one would expect a significant increase in brain-related problems. Indeed some neurological conditions support this association. According to the CDC 11 percent of all school-aged children in the United States carry a diagnosis of attention deficit hyperactivity disorder.[142] These figures are astounding when considering that the majority of these children have been prescribed toxic neuro-stimulants for treatment. If one looks carefully at the clinical criteria for ADHD (no lab or diagnostic test for the condition exists), various behaviors associated with inattention, hyperactivity, and impulsivity are required. Interestingly these reflect the same symptoms seen in children suffering from sleep deprivation. Anyone around a sleep-deprived child can verify the fact that they listen poorly, demonstrate irritability and restlessness, and often exhibit increased motor activity. Several studies have shown as many as half of children diagnosed with ADHD

---

[141] Brumfield, Ben. "Shift workers beware: Sleep loss may cause brain damage, new research says." CNN.com, 2014. Retrieved from http://www.cnn.com/2014/03/19/health/sleep-loss-brain-damage/.

[142] Thakkar, Vatsal G. "Diagnosing the wrong deficit." The New York Times, 2013. Retrieved from http://www.nytimes.com/2013/04/28/opinion/sunday/diagnosing-the-wrong-deficit.html?_r=0.

no longer demonstrate ADHD symptoms after correcting their sleep deprivation problems.[143]

Memory loss, poor learning capacity, and poor attention are perhaps among the most notable neurological effects from sleep deprivation; however, sleep deprivation also affects other health systems. Immune system dysfunction represents another major effect from inadequate sleep. Sleep can be divided into different stages based on the presence of rapid eye movement (REM) during sleep as well as the depth of sleep. During non-REM sleep, when one is in a deep sleep (also known as slow-wave sleep), several physiological changes occur that facilitate health. For children slow-wave sleep is in abundance because this sleep state prompts advanced growth and development. But even in adulthood roughly 25 percent of our sleep is slow-wave sleep, and this state augments the body's ability to fight infections, eliminate cancerous cells, and repair tissues.

In essence a reduction in the quantity of sleep results in a reduction of slow-wave sleep. In turn shifts in the number of lymphocytes and other immune cells occur, causing a weakened ability to maintain ongoing health. This condition makes individuals more prone to infections as well as cancers over time.[144] If one has ever suffered from the common cold, the need for additional sleep is quite evident (whether one chooses to get it or not). The ability to fight off viruses and bacteria depends on a well-balanced immune system, and without adequate sleep this balance is negatively affected. Recent studies in animals have also demonstrated how fragmented sleep

---

[143] Ibid.

[144] Mann, Denise. "Coping with excessive sleepiness." *WebMD*, 2010. Retrieved from http://www.webmd.com/sleep-disorders/excessive-sleepiness-10/immune-system-lack-of-sleep.

results in more aggressive and invasive tumor growth.[145] While the purpose of sleep in its totality remains poorly understood, specific T lymphocytes peak during the night when deep sleep most commonly occurs. Failure to provide the body with enough slow-wave sleep inevitably weakens the immune system's ability to function normally.

Sleep deprivation similarly alters the immune system and inflammatory proteins during the day as well as during the night. When sleep is lacking, the body becomes overly stressed and reacts through its typical stress mechanisms. In regard to the immune system, chemicals that favor inflammation are released, and these interact with stress hormonal systems to cause a variety of metabolic changes. For example, higher levels of cortisol are released with stress, which in turn enhances adrenaline-like hormone responses. Heart rate, blood pressure, and other cardiovascular changes occur gradually over time as heightened levels of stress hormones and inflammation develop.[146] This mechanism is believed to account for the increased incidence of hypertension and heart disease among sleep-deprived subjects in some studies.[147]

Other hormonal changes affecting glucose metabolism and hunger mechanisms also occur with a chronic lack of sleep. Research has shown that sleep deprivation results in lower levels of the hormone leptin (which normally suppresses appetite) and an increase in the

---

[145] Hakim, F., Wang, Y., Zhang, S.X., Zheng, J., Yolcu, E.S., Carreras, A., Khalyfa, A., Shirwan, H., Almendros, I. & Gozal, D. "Fragmented sleep accelerates tumor growth and progression through recruitment of tumor-associated macrophages and TLR4 signaling." *Cancer Research*, 2014.

[146] AlDabal, Laila, and Ahmed S. BaHammam. "Metabolic, endocrine, and immune consequences of sleep deprivation." *The Open Respiratory Medicine Journal* 5 (2011): 31-43.

[147] Ibid.

hormone ghrelin (which normally stimulates hunger). This combination along with fatigue and sleepiness results in selective choices to eat high-calorie carbohydrates and avoid physical exercise.[148] The natural consequences of these events are weight gain and increasing glucose intolerance, and indeed both obesity and diabetes are significantly increased among sleep-deprived individuals. Some research has shown that people sleeping less than six hours a night are twice as likely to develop diabetes over time compared to those sleeping more than eight hours.[149]

As can be seen, the effects of sleep deprivation on health are numerous, affecting a variety of bodily systems. Proactive approaches to this problem involve behavioral changes with commitments to get adequate rest on a daily basis. But social pressures, just like the ones I experienced in medical residency, are often too powerful to overcome without serious consequences. Without question these can be challenging situations with which to deal. Of course ideally, health-focused institutions should be relied upon to promote such policies of social change. But unfortunately this is often not the case in conventional medicine.

Conventional Approaches to Sleep Deprivation

It remains interesting that conventional medicine, which strives to promote health and wellness, fails to institute policies that favor well-being among its own medical trainees. Failing to allow medical providers adequate time to sleep can be compared to a restaurant failing to ensure its food is adequately refrigerated. Eventually something

---

[148] Ibid.
[149] Ibid.

bad will happen as a result. In fact recent statistics show that nearly 100,000 deaths result from medical errors annually, making this category the sixth leading cause of death in the United States.[150] How many of these medical errors can be attributed to sleep deprivation remains unknown, but based on the widespread prevalence of sleep deprivation among medical residents and the population at large, a significant percentage can be suspected.

Indeed conventional medicine to date has been slow to appreciate the importance of sleep on health. But over the last couple of decades the business of sleep has grown substantially. Based on recent analyses the sleep medicine industry exceeded $32.4 billion in 2012 revenues, which reflected a growth of nearly 9 percent in four years.[151] The focus, however, has not been primarily on sleep deprivation specifically or on strategies to get people to obtain needed sleep hours. In fact the majority of revenues come from costly overnight sleep studies looking for other sleep disorder causes, from sleep equipment sales for snoring and sleep apnea, and from pharmaceutical sales for insomnia. The revenue from over-the-counter sleep medications in 2007 alone was $604 million![152] Among prescription sleep aids for insomnia, nearly all have been identified as being habit-forming and addictive in nature when taken regularly. Thus once one is on such medications, reversing course becomes increasingly difficult, leading to ever-enlarging profits for drug companies. Now add in sales from

---

[150] American Association for Justice. "Preventable medical errors—The sixth biggest killer in America." Justice.org, 2014. Retrieved from http://www.justice.org/cps/rde/justice/hs.xsl/8677.htm.

[151] Mackey, Maureen. "Sleepless in America: A $32.4 billion business." The Fiscal Times, 2012. Retrieved from http://www.thefiscaltimes.com/Articles/2012/07/23/Sleepless-in-America-A-32-4-Billion-Business?page=0%2C0.

[152] Ibid.

consumer retail markets selling various energy drinks and stimulants, and the picture suddenly becomes clear.

Rather than change social behaviors and focus on the main issue of self-inflicted sleep deprivation, conventional medicine, the pharmaceutical industry, and other retailers have realized sleep deprivation is actually their golden goose. Sleep medicine specialists certainly provide an array of services of which many are needed and beneficial to long-term health. But at the same time the abuse of sleep aids, excessive sleep testing, and a shift in behaviors that replace stimulants for sleep can be seen as a move in the wrong direction. As a result health problems are worsening since the primary problem is being neglected. In order to enjoy optimal memory performance, more focused attention, and enhanced clarity of thought, adequate sleep is imperative. A chronic lack of sleep not only interferes with these abilities but also causes longstanding or permanent problems in cognitive function. Similarly immune function becomes compromised when sleep is lacking, increasing the risk of infections, cancers, and secondary hormonal effects. Ultimately these changes affect a variety of organ systems. The common underlying cause is simply a lack of sleep, but a reactive, conventional medical system fails to focus its attention in a proactive manner. Instead the traditional approach is to test, diagnose, and treat, and in the process precious resources of time, money, and services are wasted.

Consumer Solutions for Sleep Deprivation

With conventional medicine failing to address the primary problem and with social pressures demanding more from less, naturally consumer options attempt to provide quick-fix solutions for a chronically sleep-deprived nation. With little surprise about half of all Americans drink coffee, and most individuals average about three hundred milligrams of caffeine daily as a means to stay awake and energized.[153] But while coffee has grown in popularity over the last several decades, the more concerning segment in the retail world involves energy drinks and energy products. From sixteen-ounce mega-cans to smaller "energy shots," these products contain roughly three times the amount of caffeine as a cup of coffee in addition to other stimulants like taurine and sugar.[154] As a result a couple of these energy supplements each day boosts levels of alertness and deter sleepiness, allowing us to be presumably more productive.

The energy drink industry has become massive with total revenues exceeding $5 trillion worldwide. In the United States alone more than 200 million gallons of energy drinks are consumed with 5 percent of the population known to be heavy users.[155] But these solutions provide only short-term solutions to long-term problems. Energy drinks and products indeed enhance feelings of energy and alertness, but they are equally known for their energy crashes, subsequent cravings, and numerous side effects. Products that contain high amounts of sugar are notorious for energy "ups and downs." Likewise sugary drinks produce addictive cravings, encouraging repeated consumption time after time. Even energy drinks with no calories or

---

[153] Gaille, Brandon. "26 energy drink industry statistics and trends." *BrandonGaille.com*, 2013. Retrieved from http://brandongaille.com/26-energy-drink-industry-statistics-and-trends/.

[154] Gilbert, Beth. "The health risks of energy drinks." *Huffington Post*, 2012. Retrieved from http://www.huffingtonpost.com/2012/10/25/health-risks-energy-drinks_n_2009529.html.

[155] Gaille, 2013.

sugar have aspartame, which has already been described in terms of its harmful health effects.

Side effects associated with energy drinks include irritability, agitation, and a variety of gastrointestinal complaints. Additionally these products, due to their ingredients, naturally contribute to ongoing sleep deprivation, causing both insomnia and disruption of normal sleep stages and cycles.[156] So it should be of little surprise that energy drinks are self-promoting. Once one starts drinking these products, ongoing sleep deprivation as well as rebound cravings encourage continued use, often in escalating amounts. As a result individuals return to a chronically sleep-deprived state yet are now dependent on energy drinks to make it through their days. Once again a quick-fix solution proves ineffective in addressing the real underlying problem of the need for more sleep.

Some makers of energy drinks are facing lawsuits related to harmful side effects from their products. In Maryland a fourteen-year-old girl died after ingesting two cans of an energy drink with caffeine. According to medical investigators the cause of her death was due to a fatal cardiac arrhythmia.[157] Caffeine as well as these other stimulants has been shown to elevate systolic blood pressure and alter heart rhythms, increasing the risk for serious arrhythmias.[158] Therefore side effects from these consumer products can result in serious health risks for some people. While most people want immediate solutions to eliminate feelings of sleep deprivation, energy drinks are certainly

---

[156] Gilbert, 2012.

[157] Ibid.

[158] N.A. "Energy drinks linked to adverse health effects." *CNBC.com*, 2013. Retrieved from http://www.cnbc.com/id/100581965.

not the answer. Not only do their benefits in providing energy quickly fade, but they also pose risky health threats over time.

The nation as a whole suffers from a chronic sleep-deprived state. Pressures to get ahead, a prevailing sense of insufficient time, and an accelerated lifestyle all contribute to this trend. In the process health is sacrificed as memory functions become less sharp, attention less focused, and other health systems less effective. The answer isn't rocket science, nor does it lie within the common conventional medicine approaches. People simply need to get more sleep and restructure their lives accordingly. While a minority may have concurrent sleep disorders in addition to sleep deprivation, the majority do not. And energy supplements from coffee to energy drinks offer little in the way of long-term benefits and even less for better health. Fortunately the real solution is inexpensive, safe, and completely within one's control; additionally it is usually something everyone enjoys. All it takes is taking a good look at one's life patterns and a commitment to make time for adequate sleep. The "rest" will fall in place.

CHAPTER 7

The Air We Breathe

The body and mind require many vital compounds in order to function properly. Among them oxygen is perhaps the most vital since tissues deprived of oxygen rapidly deteriorate and become permanently damaged. In fact the human brain can only tolerate a lack of oxygen for a few short minutes before becoming permanently impaired to the point of coma. In contrast the brain's ability to tolerate low glucose levels is much longer. Naturally the quality of the air affects the ability to gain oxygen, and at the same time air quality presents many other potential hazards for health when it contains other substances. With increased industrialization of most nations throughout the world, air pollution has rapidly become a global concern prompting environmental changes and policies. But these changes have been notably insufficient, and many harmful compounds knowingly exist in the air today with little to no effort taken to address them.

Smog and industrial pollution have been well described in the media, and EPA guidelines and standards routinely attempt to regulate air quality in regards to common pollutants like carbon monoxide, nitrogen oxides, sulfur dioxide, and various volatile organic compounds. But what about those hidden substances in the air that escape detection or routine measurement? Aerosolized heavy metals commonly affect air quality and come from a range of sources, while vaporization of other chemicals from fire retardants and formaldehyde-containing products infect the air chronically over time. Similar to other chemicals in the environment, these agents are poorly studied, infrequently considered, and haphazardly addressed by environmental agencies, conventional health providers, and product manufacturers. The nature of symptoms caused by these compounds, combined with the costs and challenges of determining cause and effect, deters needed investigations. And in some cases, alternative motives other than health further prevent such efforts.

In this chapter poorly recognized (yet common) air pollutants will be discussed in relation to human health as well as the importance of appreciating their long-term detrimental effects. From heavy metals permeating the air in nano-sized particles to volatile compounds such as PBB and formaldehyde, different pollutants will be highlighted in terms of their increasing environmental presence and their negative effects on health. Not only will their abundance in the air we breathe be revealing, but the lack of attention in protecting the public from these compounds and the ongoing motivation to do nothing will likely be surprising.

Is It Safe Inside?

Did you know Americans spend more than 90 percent of their time indoors? Think about it. From the hours people sleep, watch television, and prepare and eat meals to their occupations indoors, this statistic is easy to accept. But did you also know the number of indoor pollutants are on average five times higher than outdoor pollutants? In some cases indoor pollutants can reach one hundred times the amount of outdoor pollutants.[159] According to the EPA common indoor pollutants come from building materials, room furnishings, cleaning materials, personal care products, heating and air conditioning systems, and pesticide applications. In addition external toxins such as radon and outdoor pollutants can also routinely invade indoor space.[160] In essence the higher concentration of pollutants in the air within a dwelling occurs because toxins become trapped inside, thus exposing individuals to higher volumes of pollutants over time.

My first known experience with indoor air pollutants occurred in 1980, shortly after making the decision to attend medical school. The buildings on campus where I attended school were undergoing extensive renovations, and naturally some building materials were being destroyed while new ones were being constructed. Within weeks I began feeling fatigued, anxious, and unable to concentrate. Despite having made straight A's in college, including courses like organic chemistry, I struggled to make a passing grade that first year. And despite being a trained cellist in the Alabama Symphony, I found it challenging to stay active, social, and engaged in extracurricular interests. Even my personality seemed to be changing with feelings of nervousness, paranoia, and a desire to be left alone. Not knowing the cause of my complaints, I became increasingly perplexed.

However, one day while in gross anatomy class, I had the revelation. Amid all the cadavers that were used for dissection and anatomy education, I noticed a worsening of my complaints as the smell of

---

[159] EPA. "Buildings and their impact on the environment: A statistical summary." *Environmental Protection Agency Green Building,* 2009. Retrieved from http://www.epa.gov/greenbuilding/pubs/gbstats.pdf.
[160] Ibid.

formaldehyde permeated the room. This observation, and later information revealing formaldehyde as a common source of "sick building
syndrome," identified the primary culprit for my abrupt changes. As I
later found out, this exposure to this particular indoor pollutant was
just one of several toxins that affected my cognitive, psychological,
and physical health. However, the chemicals released into the air from
the construction renovations and from the lab clearly contributed to
my difficulties academically and socially.

Sick building syndrome is a well-recognized condition affecting
thousands of individuals annually. Symptoms often involve headaches, irritation of the eyes and nose, itchiness, dizziness, nausea,
reduced concentration, fatigue, and odor sensitivity.[161] These symptoms are naturally associated with reduced levels of performance and
productivity. One of the defining features of sick building syndrome
is that a known trigger fails to exist (which seems rather backward)
and that symptoms are consistently associated with being in the
building.[162]

Despite the diagnosis of sick building syndrome failing to identify
a single cause or conglomeration of causes, various indoor toxins are
readily accepted as being potential sources of the condition. Indoor
pollutants from adhesives, paints, upholstery, carpeting, wood products, cleaning agents, and more are identified as potential causative
agents in addition to biological contaminants like bacteria, viruses,
molds, and fungi. Among the most likely toxins causing sick building syndrome are volatile organic compounds or VOCs. This group

---

[161] National Safety Council. "Sick building syndrome." *National Safety Council*, 2009.
Retrieved from http://www.nsc.org/news_resources/Resources/Documents/Sick_
Building_Syndrome.pdf.
[162] Ibid.

of substances are chemicals in the aforementioned products, which easily evaporate into the air at room temperature (hence the term "volatile"). Examples of VOCs include formaldehyde, perchloroethylene, methylene, vinyl chloride, and more. While these substances may not sound familiar, they are certainly ever-present within most households. In fact fifty to a hundred VOCs are typically present in a single home at any one time.[163] The higher number of such products and VOCs within the home, the poorer the indoor air quality is likely to be.

Formaldehyde has been discussed in previous chapters as a toxin to human health. Its presence in some vaccines and as a metabolite of aspartame highlighted how it can negatively affect health on a regular basis through immunizations and diet. But additionally formaldehyde is present as a VOC in many glues, resins, carpets, and wood products. And though the smell may not be as apparent as in the gross anatomy lab, its health effects can still be profound. Recognized as a carcinogen, formaldehyde affects several different organ systems with nasopharyngeal cancers, brain malignancies, and leukemias, representing long-term cancer risks.[164] And as a neurotoxin, formaldehyde affects memory, energy levels, concentration, and personality.[165]

In addition to personal experience from formaldehyde exposure through allergy shots, immunizations, and building-related VOCs, I also was exposed to another VOC under the name of polybrominated

---

[163] Peltier, Karen. "Volatile Organic Compounds (VOCs): What they're all about." *About.com*. Retrieved from http://greencleaning.about.com/od/GreenCleaning Resources/g/Volatile-Organic-Compounds-Vocs-What-They-Re-All-About.htm.

[164] National Cancer Institute. "Formaldehyde and cancer risk." *National Cancer Institute*, 2012. Retrieved from http://www.cancer.gov/cancertopics/factsheet/Risk/formaldehyde.

[165] Ibid.

biphenyls or PBB. PBB is a manmade chemical used as a flame-retardant found in many plastics today. In fact it has been in use since the early 1970s. As luck would have it (bad luck that is), I grew up in Dearborn, Michigan, where one of the largest PBB contaminations ever occurred. In 1973 approximately twenty bags of PBB were mistakenly sent in bags labeled as magnesium oxide, which was normally used as a cattle feed supplement. As a result thousands of livestock received PBB, subsequently contaminating numerous agricultural products including eggs, dairy products, and meats. By the time the accident had been realized more than a year later, populations in the lower portions of Michigan and some surrounding states had been exposed to large quantities of PBB.[166]

Environmental agencies subsequently quarantined five hundred farms, including thirty thousand cattle, forty-five hundred swine, 1.5 million chickens as well as millions of grocery store products, but the damage had already been done. A method to remove PBB from the body has not been well established, and the chemical's half-life exceeds ten years, meaning the chemical persists for more than half a century in one's body.[167] Having now been tested for PBB, I can verify that the chemical indeed hangs around for a long time and in significant amounts. The estimated exposure to the inhabitants of Michigan at that time was twenty times higher than the rate of normal exposure, and subsequent observations demonstrated significant health effects PBB can cause.

Immediate symptoms from PBB included nausea, fatigue, rashes,

---

[166] Michigan Department of Community Health. "PBBs (Polybrominated Biphenyls) in Michigan." *MDCH*, 2011. Retrieved from http://www.michigan.gov/documents/mdch_PBB_FAQ_92051_7.pdf.

[167] Ibid.

muscle aches, and general malaise as many farmers complained of these problems, prompting the initial investigations. Subsequently PBB has been found to have significant effects on the endocrine and reproductive systems, and likewise it has been recognized as a likely carcinogen. In addition to increased abortion rates and menstrual disturbances, increased rates of liver cancer, breast cancer, gastrointestinal cancers, and lymphomas have been recorded among those affected.[168] Despite these definitive findings the EPA does not regulate the amount of PBB in plastics or the amount of PBB in households in the United States. In fact, with the exception of formaldehyde, which is monitored loosely in some residential settings, none of the VOCs is regulated by the EPA or housing authorities.[169] This lack of attention persists despite findings that indoor levels of VOCs and other pollutants far exceed those outdoors. In order to combat these hidden indoor pollutants, the use of HEPA filters (high-efficiency particulate air) is an effective means by which indoor air quality can be significantly improved.

Hidden Threats Outdoors

Most people presume to be well-informed about outdoor air pollution. Amid frequent news reports of global climate change and increasing greenhouse gas emissions, knowledge of harmful gases in the air like carbon monoxide, carbon dioxide, and nitrogen compounds seems to be common. To a great extent the EPA and other environmental

---

[168] Ibid.

[169] Greenguard Certification. "Indoor air quality: Chemicals." *Greenguard.org*, 2014. Retrieved from http://www.greenguard.org/en/indoorAirQuality/iaq_chemicals.aspx.

agencies promote such awareness in an effort to change societal behaviors and to justify their regulatory actions. And indeed these gases
and toxins clearly represent harmful substances to human health.
But is the extent of knowledge about outdoor air pollution really
that comprehensive? And has the full story about air pollution been
completely revealed?

Outdoor air pollution comes from many sources. Combustion
of fossil fuels for energy accounts for a significant source as do industrial byproducts. Likewise the transportation sector accounts for
many pollutants not only from energy production but also from aerosolized particles coming from tires, roadways, and other structures.
Even farming industries contribute to air pollution through biomass
wastes and ammonia gas production.[170] Each of these sources of air
pollution are referred to as primary pollutants since they originate
from human sources of activity. And certainly these are important
sources of pollution.

In addition to these primary sources, however, secondary sources
of air pollution also exist. These occur when primary pollutants interact. Similar to the unknown effects resulting from the combined use
of pesticides, pollutants can combine to create new and unknown pollutant effects. Likewise these new combinations affect human health
in ways that often exceed a laboratory's capabilities in detection.[171]
One of the best-known secondary pollutants is ozone, which develops
when common primary air pollutants are exposed to sunlight. Ozone
is the brown smog that plagues many urban areas, especially in the hot

---

[170] European Lung Foundation. "Outdoor air pollution: Air quality and health."
EuropeanLungFoundation.org, n.d. Retrieved from http://www.european-lung-
foundation.org/126-european-lung-foundation-elf-outdoor-air-pollution.htm.
[171] Ibid.

summer. Without a doubt this secondary pollutant has dramatically increased rates of many respiratory diseases including asthma, pneumonia, and lung cancer.[172] But while the effects of ozone are partially appreciated, the effects of many other secondary pollutants are not.

According to environmental studies in Europe, more than 455,000 premature deaths occur in Europe each year due to outdoor air pollutants. These deaths are primarily related to pulmonary and cardiovascular effects of these chemicals.[173] Usually air pollution is rarely identified as the primary culprit in an individual's illness, and even when mass population data is considered, air pollution from vehicles, industries, and farms is blamed as the primary problem. Interestingly while these sources of pollution are very real and important, many other sources of outdoor air pollution exist and are much more intentional in nature. But rarely will these sources of outdoor air pollution be cited as being problematic or even existing.

Ever looked into the sky and seen a speeding jet leave behind a stream of white clouds? Ever seen several jets at once leaving behind a checkerboard pattern of lines that then gradually expand, creating a diffuse opaque film? If so, you are not alone. In all likelihood these patterns represent what are known as "chemtrails." Chemtrails are essentially trails of aerosolized chemicals emitted from jets that pollute the skies and then contaminate the air we breathe. But these chemicals are not simply fuel exhaust. Instead these chemicals represent various heavy metals compounds and gases that are intentionally released in order to affect the environment. Also known as stratospheric aerosol geo-engineering, chemtrails are used to modify weather patterns or affect climate change. In other instances militaries and governments

---

[172] Ibid.
[173] Ibid.

may possibly pollute the skies with chemtrails for more concerning purposes like chemical warfare and depopulation efforts.[174] These are sources of outdoor air pollution about which relatively few people know or talk.

In defense of chemtrails, many experts and state officials deny their existence, indicating that these white streaks in the sky are simply "contrails," or condensation trails, which result from normal jet exhaust. But even government militaries have admitted to the use of chemtrails. In 1997 the US Air Force reported spreading two million seven-ounce bundles of aerosolized aluminum (known as CHAFF) in various locations. And in 2002 the US Navy reported dropping hundreds of thousands of pounds of CHAFF around the Chesapeake Bay area.[175] Groups in the United States, Canada, Australia, and New Zealand had consistently reported the presence of chemtrails in their countries.[176] Based on this information it seems unlikely that chemtrails are simply figments of a paranoid imagination.

Common chemicals released in chemtrail emissions include nano-sized aluminum particles, barium, strontium, and radioactive thorium. CHAFF specifically is nano-sized aluminum-coated fiberglass.[177] These agents are released into the atmosphere in aerosolized forms and persist in the air for long periods of time. However, they eventually settle onto the ground and in water supplies. So unlike

---

[174] Swinney, Clare. "Declassified NZ Defense Force reports reveal chemtrail linked to outbreak of illnesses." InfoNews.co.nz, 2011. Retrieved from http://infonews.co.nz/news.cfm?id=62532.

[175] Perlingieri, Ilya Sandra. "Chemtrails: The consequences of toxic metals and chemical aerosols on human health." GlobalResearch.org, 2014. Retrieved from http://www.globalresearch.ca/chemtrails-the-consequences-of-toxic-metals-and-chemical-aerosols-on-human-health/19047.

[176] Ibid.

[177] Ibid.

contrails, which rapidly disappear, chemtrails remain much longer and gradually permeate not only the air we breathe but also the entire environment.

The negative health effects from aluminum have been described previously and include memory loss, irritability, reduced alertness, and personality changes. In addition to these effects, aerosolized heavy metals also cause other conditions like asthma, pneumonia, flu-like complaints, and heart disease.[178] Based on these discoveries it's no wonder that millions of deaths worldwide occur as a result of air pollution.

Common knowledge about air pollution today is provided through mainstream sources like the media and government agencies. Sustainability issues concerning the environment draw a great deal of attention (as they should) about the more common air pollutants derived from cars, factories, and farming. But many other indoor and outdoor air pollutants exist and are significant in quantity and effect. Chemicals like VOCs and fire retardants permeate the indoor air, where many spend more than 90 percent of their time. And even outside in remote locations where urban smog is supposed to be non-existent, chemicals pumped into the stratosphere still contaminate the surroundings. Unfortunately common sources of information provide very little insights into these health risks.

Without greater transparency and more comprehensive knowledge, the ability to recognize these threats to human health are certainly challenging. Yet the telltale signs are ever-present. Asthma continues to be a serious health problem among children as well as adults, and the rates of respiratory and cardiovascular disease remain

---

[178] Ibid.

tremendously high despite advances in conventional medicine. These phenomena reveal that the underlying source of the problem remains and that secondarily addressing the damage once it has occurred offers a poor strategy for better health. Air quality is essential to good health. Knowing both the visible and invisible air pollutants present is the first step (in addition to their reasons for being there in the first place!) so that elimination of these substances can then be pursued. Only once this knowledge is gained can preventative steps leading to better health be achieved.

CHAPTER 8

Other Invisible Health Threats: EMR

According to recent global statistics, enough mobile device subscriptions have now been sold to support 96 percent of the world's population. In 2013 more than 6.8 billion mobile technology subscriptions had been realized, representing a significant increase from the 5.4 billion recorded in 2010.[179] Such a figure is hard to image when one considers that mobile technologies hardly existed a few decades ago. Similar increases have occurred in personal computers of course, and now all sorts of objects will soon be able to communicate with each other. A refrigerator will be able to send notifications alerting consumers that only a couple of eggs are left in the container or that the milk will expire in two days. With the "Internet of things," the information age will take yet another huge step forward…or perhaps backwards

Increasingly the world is becoming saturated with electrical and magnetic signals that allow wireless and remote objects to communicate. This comes as no surprise since the human body itself is

---

[179] N.A. "Global mobile statistics 2014 Part A: Mobile subscribers; handset market share; mobile operators." *MobiThinking.com*, 2014. Retrieved from http://mobithinking.com/mobile-marketing-tools/latest-mobile-stats/a.

composed of millions of cells that rely on cellular mechanisms based on positive and negative electrical charges. Energy production, cell metabolism, and electrolyte balance all use electrical charges to function normally. And each of these is important in how well the immune system, hormonal system, and other systems operate daily. But what is lacking is a detailed awareness of how these two things collide. In other words how well can the human body function when it becomes bombarded with environmental electromagnetic fields?

In this chapter the effects of extrinsic electromagnetic radiation (EMR) sources will be discussed in addition to current evidence regarding their effects on human health. While various health and government agencies insist such exposures are completely safe, growing research suggests quite the opposite. In fact EMR may be responsible for some of today's toughest health problems, including cancer, autism, and attention deficit disorder. A medical condition labeled "electromagnetic hypersensitivity" has even been identified for many exposed to low levels of EMR over long periods of time.[180] Not only must preventative health care consider the air we breathe, the water we drink, and the food we eat. It must also consider the silent and invisible threats that surround us every day.

Defining the Scope of EMR Exposure

Electricity deals with voltage. The greater the voltage, the greater the amount of electricity. Magnetic fields on the other hand deal with the flow of electricity. Instead of varying with voltage, magnetic

---

[180] Rees, Camilla. "Biological effects of electromagnetic fields." *International Institute for Building-Biology & Ecology: Healthy Bodies Healthy Buildings Conference 2012.* Retrieved from http://www.youtube.com/watch?v=Z88glpsehQY.

fields vary with the amount of electricity consumed since this reflects the amount of electricity flowing from one point to another. When electricity flows, an electromagnetic field (EMF) is created, and from these fields electromagnetic radiations spread. Of course these EMRs cannot be seen and oftentimes can be difficult to measure, but regardless they are ever-present and represent invisible and silent forces throughout our environments.

EMFs occur naturally as well. The reason a compass can be used to determine directionality reflects the EMF created from the earth's flow of electrical energy from one pole to the other. Thunderstorms and atmospheric EMFs are certainly common, accounting for a variety of weather patterns and effects. And the human body, as mentioned, is composed of thousands of tiny EMFs at a cellular and tissue level. Brain and nervous system tissues in particular depend on these fields in order to conduct nerve impulses and to function normally. But at the same time manmade inventions are accounting for an increasing amount of EMFs within the world, and like greenhouse gas emissions, questions about their long-term effects on human and environmental health are being raised.

EMFs differ in their strengths. Those with shorter wavelengths carry higher amounts of energy and are potentially more damaging. Such fields emit ionizing EMR, which indicates the EMR energy is powerful enough to break existing molecular bonds. EMRs such as gamma rays, x-rays, and cosmic rays are examples of ionizing radiation, and their detrimental effects on health and human tissues have been known for some time.[181] But what is less well known are the effects of chronic exposure to lower energy EMR on health. This

[181] World Health Organization. "What are electromagnetic fields?" *WHO.Int*, 2014. Retrieved from http://www.who.int/peh-emf/about/WhatisEMF/en/index1.html.

non-ionizing EMR has been reported to be quite safe, but increasingly evidence is suggesting otherwise.

Low levels of non-ionizing radiation come from a host of objects in the world today. Power lines, microwaves, computers, televisions, cellular phones, and cell phone towers represent some of the more common sources of low-level EMR. The strength of these fields are indeed low, but the growth in number of these devices and structures is rapidly increasing the density of these EMFs. A recent report that assessed urban city schools throughout the United States found that schools in ten state capitals were within a quarter mile of one hundred or more antennas. Likewise the report stated that 63 percent of American students, or 1.4 million children in total, were at risk for exposure to microwave radiation as a result of nearby antennas.[182]

These figures demonstrate the widespread presence of electromagnetic radiation throughout the world today. As technologies have advanced, the number of EMR fields have likewise grown. From household electrical outlets to neighborhood cell phone towers, EMR surrounds human existence. Therefore the issue of exposure is not something in need of investigation since nearly everyone is being exposed to some degree. Instead the important questions pertain to the level of EMRs needed to negatively affect human health. If high-energy EMR can cause damage over short periods of time by damaging molecular bonds then couldn't low-energy EMR similarly cause comparable damage given more time?

---

[182] Hagas, Mavda. "BRAG antenna ranking of schools." *Electromagnetichealth. org*, 2010. Retrieved from http://electromagnetichealth.org/wp-content/uploads/2010/04/BRAG_Schools.pdf.

EMR and Health

The association between EMR and negative health effects is not something new. In fact some evidence of these effects dates back nearly a century. Epidemiological studies conducted in the first half of the twentieth century explored the rapidly increasing rate of acute lymphocytic leukemia in children in Great Britain and in the United States. After exploring a variety of potential causes, the prevalence of residential electrification of homes in both countries was found to best correlate with these increases. Between 1911 and 1920 leukemia mortality rates among children increased by 4.5 percent per year, and this increase paralleled the rate at which homes were being constructed with routine electrical wiring and outlets. This report out of the Washington State Department of Health suggested that 75 percent of all acute lymphocytic leukemias were attributable to residential electrification, and that as many as 60 percent of all childhood leukemias were likely preventable.[183]

Fast forward to today. More than two million cell phone towers exist in the United States alone. Every home not only has electricity but computers, televisions, microwaves, and a range of appliances, all of which increase EMR. Between 2003 and 2007 EMR exponentially increased by a factor of one quadrillion![184] So if negative health effects were realized as early as 1920 from EMR, just imagine the potential health effects it is causing today. Evidence now exists that

---

[183] Milham, S., and E. M. Ossiander. "Historical evidence that residential electrification caused the emergence of the childhood leukemia peak." *Medical Hypotheses* 56, no. 3 (2001): 290-295.

[184] Greene, Deborah. "EMF radiation dangers and protection." *YourEnergyMatters. com*, 2011. Retrieved from http://debragreene.com/radiation.asp.

the rise in EMR parallels the rapidly increasing prevalence of autism and attention deficit disorder. Even the World Health Organization recognizes microwave radiation frequencies as carcinogenic.[185] And a condition now known as electromagnetic hypersensitivity syndrome (EHS) has been identified as resulting from chronic low levels of EMR exposure.[186]

Interestingly the first description of EHS occurred in the 1950s in the Soviet Union. Under the name of radiofrequency radiation sickness, researchers identified a variety of symptoms commonly associated with low-level radiofrequency radiation exposure over a prolonged period of time. Symptoms included headache, fatigue, ocular dysfunction, sleep impairment, and dizziness. Likewise skin-related problems were often present, which included eczema, psoriasis, or allergic dermatitis.[187] Other researchers have since found similar constellations of symptoms under the label of EHS. Skin reactions can involve redness, tingling, or burning, and other complaints can include fatigue, reduced concentration, dizziness, nausea and indigestion.[188] Even the World Health Organization (WHO) has recognized this syndrome under the name of idiopathic environmental intolerance. While WHO is reluctant to conclude that this condition is caused by

---

[185] Foster, Susan D. "WHO knew about harm from electromagnetic radiation." *InfoWars.com*, 2014. Retrieved from http://www.infowars.com/who-knew-about-harm-from-electromagnetic-radiation/.

[186] Rees, 2012.

[187] Levitt, B. Blake, and Henry Lai. "Biological effects from exposure to electromagnetic radiation emitted by cell tower base stations and other antenna arrays." *Environmental Reviews* 18, no. NA (2010): 369-395.

[188] Ibid.

EMFs, it does conclude the syndrome is real and affects between 2 and 3 percent of the population in many nations around the world.[189]

While numerous studies have been performed to assess the acute toxicity related to EMR exposure, very few studies examine the effects of long-term, low-level exposure. For acute exposures, thermal mechanisms are thought to play a more important role in causing biological injury. However, in long-term, low-level exposures, non-thermal mechanisms are believed to be more relevant. Indeed a review of all available studies involving low-level EMR exposure identifies several non-thermal mechanisms by which EMR causes harm to the body.[190] Animal research has supported that low-level EMR causes increased DNA damage, reduced DNA repair mechanisms, increased cellular influx of calcium, and increased permeability of the protective blood-brain barrier.[191] Based on these potential mechanisms, numerous organ systems could be affected by such exposure.

The adverse effects on health from low-level EMR have been examined through epidemiological studies as well. The results of these studies have shown specifically that adult and child leukemias, brain tumors, and other cancers have a higher incidence for individuals living near broadcast towers or having increased EMR exposure. Additionally, sleep disturbances, elevations in blood pressure, headaches, and dizziness are also more common.[192] Neurological effects portray some of the more profound symptoms and involve reduced

---

[189] World Health Organization. "Electromagnetic Hypersensitivity." *Proceedings International Workshop on EMF Hypersensitivity, Prague, Czech Republic, 2006.* Retrieved from http://www.who.int/peh-emf/publications/reports/EHS Proceedings June2006.pdf.

[190] Levitt, 2010.

[191] Ibid.

[192] Ibid.

memory and concentration and mental health impairments as well as tremors. Lastly, immune system and reproductive system effects have also been demonstrated through research studies.[193] However, despite this scientific evidence supporting the negative health effects of low-level EMR, resistance and denial in attributing these complaints to EMFs still persists.

As noted, some recognition that EMR is carcinogenic has occurred. In the United States, the specific absorption rate (the rate at which the human body may absorb energy) deemed to be safe for human health has been established as EMR exposure at 1.6 W/kg per one gram of tissue or less. While this figure is not important to memorize, comparing this value to the SAR value in the literature causing EHS and EMR-related symptoms is noteworthy. This safe upper limit SAR value on average in studies examining low-level EMR effects was significantly lower at 0.022 W/kg.[194] Because the United States as well as other nations only acknowledges the acute (thermal) effects of EMR exposure, long-term effects of low-level EMR are ignored. Therefore what government policies view as safe levels of EMR is well beyond what actually may be safe. So if avoidance of EMR exposure is going to occur, it appears individuals will have to take measures into their own hands.

Efforts to Protect Yourself from EMR Exposure

Attempts to completely avoid EMFs and EMR are no longer possible within the world in which we live. From appliances to computers to cell phone towers, such macro and micro EMFs are ever-present. But

---

[193] Ibid.
[194] Ibid.

this does mean avoiding exposure and utilizing preventative measures to reduce EMR "load" should not be tried. Like most toxins, EMR is dose-dependent; in other words the greater amount of exposure directly correlates with the risk for negative health effects. Therefore each of us can take measures to prevent illness through protective efforts.

Some efforts utilize basic common sense. Because EMFs and EMR are enhanced when connected to electrical networks, disconnecting unused appliances and electrical devices serves to reduce EMR exposure. For example, unplugging computers and other chargeable items once fully charged reduces the constant electrical impulse flowing to these pieces of equipment. Likewise if wireless routers need to be used, isolating these devices in small, unused rooms is ideal. If possible, avoiding such Wi-Fi networks and instead hardwiring connections can be of even greater benefit. Similarly, disconnecting Bluetooth and other roaming connection software reduces the near-continuous electromagnetic fields created by these signal-searching devices.[195] In essence the goal in reducing EMF and EMR exposure is simply to "unplug" as many electrical components as possible to minimize the radiofrequency and electromagnetic signals surrounding us.

One of the most detrimental forms of low-level EMR comes from "transients." Transients describe electrical activity that has nearly continuous and repeated electrical current interruptions. Transients are most common in energy-efficient devices. In order to reduce energy utilization, these devices turn on and off thousands of times per second, but at the same time these repeated current interruptions

---

[195] Lipman, Frank. "13 ways to protect yourself from electromagnetic radiation." *DrFrankLipman.com*, 2013. Retrieved from http://www.drfranklipman. com/13-ways-to-protect-yourself-from-electromagnetic-radiation/.

stimulate what has become known as "dirty electricity." Transients create EMR pollution in our environments, which has an even greater potential to negatively affect health.[196] Components that create significant amounts of transients often have transformers and ballasts on their power cords or within their casing. Common household items that fall into this category include light dimmer switches, compact fluorescent bulbs, computers, printers, and cell phones.[197] Minimizing these devices in the home and/or disconnecting them once charged greatly reduces EMR exposure.

Reducing EMR exposure through the aforementioned behaviors is important but far from complete. EMFs are ubiquitous, and therefore more active measures may be needed if one lives in an EMF-heavy location or if one is sensitive to the effects of EMR and has EHS. In these instances, choosing to use electromagnetic-blocking technology offers an additional solution. These products, which include specialized clothing, bracelets, necklaces, and pendants, offer different approaches to reducing EMR exposure. Some create their own electromagnetic frequencies that are known to better parallel biological systems. In this way they augment normal, healthy physiological functioning of the body, reducing other potentially harmful external influences from local EMFs. Other products instead "block" these external EMFs through lined fabrics and coverings that shield one from EMF radiations. Many of these products use copper, silver, and/or nickel as the shielding material.

Of particular importance is one's bedroom. Sleep quality is

---

[196] Segell, Michael. "Is dirty electricity making you sick?" *Prevention*, 2011. Retrieved from http://www.prevention.com/health/healthy-living/electromagnetic-fields-and-your-health.
[197] Ibid.

affected in the majority of people with EHS, and EMR is associated with reductions in melatonin as well as other hormonal disruptions.[198] EMR-shielded canopies for beds are available as are covers for digital clocks. These products, along with active EMR blockers or shields, can reduce EHS symptoms as well as reduce health risks during sleep. These products allow one's immune system to function optimally and in turn reduce cancer risk as well as other systemic problems. For me personally, I utilize a pendant product designed to enhance normal biorhythms and natural physiological EMFs. As a result the potential effects from other environmental EMFs are nullified.

In summary, proactive individuals recognizing harmful environmental effects from EMFs will employ avoidance techniques and actively pursue measures to protect their health. Minimizing exposure to EMFs in the home, workplace, and other locations can serve to reduce the overall EMR dose received over time and thus reduce health risks. And active measures involving blocking or shielding products further protect normal biologic processes, allowing the body to function normally. Complete elimination of EMR is neither possible nor necessary, but keeping one's exposure to a minimum is important in an effort to maintain optimal health and deter the array of illnesses clearly associated with EMR.

As is often the case with many environmental toxins, a long latency period between exposure and disease occurrence interferes with the ability to define cause and effect with 100-percent accuracy for some time. Exposure to asbestos, for example, was not initially known to cause lung disease until many years later when thousands of workers had been exposed. The same could be said of chemicals

---

[198] Levitt, 2010.

like diethylstilbestrol, which is now known to cause serious birth defects. In considering EMR and health effects, this problem is magnified even greater. For one, the explosion of wireless networks and technological devices (including the cell phone) has occurred over a relatively brief timespan. Therefore, enough time has not yet lapsed to definitively prove the etiologic relationship between EMR and disease. Secondly, the invisible nature of EMR and lack of awareness of EMF density hinders most people's ability to measure exposure. For these reasons, a great deal of denial and ignorance about EMR health effects exist.

With a better appreciation of EMR and its effects on health, the ability to reduce exposure and to actively protect oneself from harm is possible. Individuals who suffer from the symptoms described in this chapter may for the first time have some insight into the potential cause of their problems. Despite awareness that such effects can be caused by EMR since the 1950s, knowledge of EMR and EHS remains poorly publicized. Even today with an abundance of evidence to the contrary, mainstream health organizations continue to downplay health problems related to EMR. By taking control of one's own health and by appreciating the information readily available, one can greatly reduce the unfortunate side effects of EMR.

CHAPTER 9

Making a Change to Pursue Real Health

By superficially examining the facts, many researchers and epidemiologists conclude that conventional medicine has made great strides over the last century. At the beginning of the twentieth century, life expectancy was between forty-five and fifty-five years on average, but by the end of the century this figure had climbed to seventy-five years. In addition to life expectancy increasing by 56 percent, the age-adjusted death rate in the United States also fell by 74 percent.[199] Clearly conventional medicine, which gained its foundations and momentum during these decades, had to be the primary force behind these favorable figures.

To be fair, conventional medicine indeed had a great deal to do with these improvements in overall health and quality of life. In 1900 a quarter of all deaths were related to infectious diseases. The discovery of bacteria and subsequently antibiotics dramatically reduced the mortality rate from these disorders. But at the same time epidemiological discoveries and changes in public health also were responsible for these improvements. Improved hygiene, clean water systems, and

---

[199] Lopez, Alan D. "Morbidity and mortality, changing patterns in the twentieth century." *Encyclopedia of biostatistics* (1998).

improvements in preventative measures also occurred during this time.[200] Therefore while conventional remedies of care advanced and included antibiotics, immunizations, and other medication and surgical therapies, so did a slow but steady trend toward prevention of disease and preservation of health.

Today the landscape is much different. Instead of infections, a variety of complex chronic and degenerative diseases tops the list of common health disorders. At the end of the twentieth century, leading causes of death included heart disease, cancer, stroke, COPD, and accidents.[201] At the same time other complex disorders like diabetes, obesity, autism, attention deficit disorder, and organ failure have become increasingly prevalent. Unlike infectious diseases that require identification of the offending organism and matching a single treatment against this agent, today's complex disorders have many risk factors and involve numerous bodily systems demanding more involved (and expensive) therapies. And though industrialized nations like the United States claim to have the best medical care in the world, statistics support that we spend over twice as much for declining levels of healthcare.[202]

Unfortunately many of the answers to today's health problems are less than straightforward, but as noted in the previous chapters, many environmental toxins and other environmental exposures play a significant part in many of these complicated diseases and illnesses.

---

[200] De Flora, Silvio, Alberto Quaglia, Carlo Bennicelli, and Marina Vercelli. "The epidemiological revolution of the 20th century." *The FASEB journal* 19, no. 8 (2005): 892-897.

[201] Lopez, 1998.

[202] Auerbach, David I., and Arthur L. Kellermann. "A decade of health care cost growth has wiped out real income gains for an average US family." *Health Affairs* 30, no. 9 (2011): 1630-1636.

Reactive, curative healthcare no longer efficiently or effectively addresses these problems. But the ability to see shortcomings in this approach has been stymied by disincentives and an inherent resistance to change. The time has come to take a fresh look at the approach to healthcare and pursue more efficient and effective methods. In this chapter exploring why this is important and how one should proceed will be discussed. Through enhanced knowledge, one can choose more wisely the best approach to optimal health. Based on the evidence, continuing to adopt conventional healthcare approaches is not likely the best option.

Rethinking Conventional Medicine

As mentioned, my father is currently ninety-seven years of age and is in remarkable health. Born in 1918, he has lived through many societal changes ranging from the Great Depression, World War II, and the Cold War to our current technological revolution. When he was a young man, industrialization had begun to boom, and these changes would eventually lead to marked advances in quality of living, or so it seemed. The number of automobiles progressively increased. Home construction soared. And eventually trends toward urbanization and globalization ensued. The amenities that individuals and families now seemed to enjoy supported advanced living, but at the same time air, water, and other forms of environmental pollution become increasingly evident. My father as a young man had little exposure to pollutants, chemicals, and pharmaceuticals, but as he aged these factors played an increasingly growing role in the overall environment.

As these changes occurred, conventional medicine gained its footing within American culture. Based on scientific theory, conventional medicine sought to apply the field of science to healthcare, which has allowed an objective approach to disease and illness prevention and treatment. But at the same time conventional medicine embraced the commercial and capitalistic structure of the American way. Skilled services received greater compensation among physicians, newer medications were naturally higher in price, and volume of care paid better than quality of care in most instances. With these incentives in place, conventional medicine naturally sought to invest in advanced technologies, pharmaceuticals, and skillsets. As the bank robber replied in response to why he robbed the bank: that's where the money is.

These comments are not meant to suggest conventional healthcare providers have conscious intentions to exploit their patients for their own personal gain. But providers, hospitals, and pharmaceutical companies are in business. Income must exceed costs, and time invested must return a yield deemed worthy of its value. Spending up to an hour educating each patient on lifestyle changes, alternative options of care, and underlying psychological motivations offers much less value (monetarily and perceptually) in comparison to a five-minute exam that produces a prescription, lab testing, and a referral to another provider. Anti-aging specialists routinely average an hour discussing health issues with their patients in comparison to conventional doctors, who often spend five minutes. In fact conventional doctors often see forty to fifty patients in a day! Besides, healthcare consumers in America have come to expect a "quick fix" to their complaints, and medication prescriptions or surgery offer a mutually pleasing option.

Conventional medicine, therefore, did not initially strive to exploit the American consumer by providing less-than-optimal care.

Instead conventional medicine simply became a product of its own environment and culture. The strides made in medications, research, surgery, and other areas support a valid attempt to provide high-quality care. However, as time progressed the healthcare machine became excessively large and powerful. The ability to perceive alternative views of disease and healthcare increasingly declined as traditional methods became deeply entrenched in the culture. Even today in the face of increasing scientific support, resistance and denial of alternative healthcare solutions persist.

Eventually even those who blindly support traditional medicine must face the facts. The United States today spends nearly $3 trillion on healthcare, which represents almost 18 percent of the gross domestic product.[203] This equates to nearly nine thousand dollars spent per person each year for healthcare services. But what do we get in return? One would assume topnotch healthcare and quality of life. However, world rankings fail to support this, and millions lack the proper access to healthcare services in this country.[204] Thus while the healthcare industry continues to turn massive profits, the overall health of the country fails to improve. Despite having some of the world's most advanced technologies, this country has an overall quality of life and life expectancy that are far from those expected of the world's best healthcare systems. How can this be?

Three main reasons account for these phenomena regarding the US healthcare system as it stands today. First, conventional medicine

---

[203] Centers for Medicare and Medicaid Services (CMS). "National health expenditures 2012 highlights." *CMS.gov*, 2013. Retrieved from http://www.cms.gov/Research-Statistics-Data-and-Systems/Statistics-Trends-and-Reports/NationalHealthExpendData/downloads/highlights.pdf.

[204] The World Bank. "Data: Health expenditure, total of GDP." WorldBank.org, 2014. Retrieved from http://data.worldbank.org/indicator/SH.XPD.TOTL.ZS.

is predominantly reactive and not proactive. Services are requested and administered when health problems develop in most cases. Instead of a focus on prevention, attention is placed on identifying and fixing existing problems. This approach is not only inefficient and costly but fails to render optimal healthcare. After all, an ounce of prevention is indeed worth a pound of cure.

Secondly, conventional medicine ignores many environmental toxins and conditions that affect health negatively. Consistently, traditional providers discount the effects of chemicals, pesticides, insecticides, hormones, and other agents used in industrialized societies. This refusal to accept such etiologies of disease stems from a need to have cause and effect scientifically proven to a high degree of certainty before considering new options. While science and scientific theory is indeed valuable, using these measures to develop a state of closed-mindedness limits the potential to explore alternative causes and treatments. And in this case, this state of mind limits the ability to move from a reactive approach to a preventative one.

The problem with conventional medicine lies within its inherent approach. In fact the traditional approach is completely backward! Currently various medicines, chemicals, and other social practices are considered safe until proven otherwise. Certainly some cursory measures to test safety are performed, but these tests are for limited amounts of time and fail to consider combination of effects. In actuality the complete opposite approach should be taken. A chemical, drug, or unnatural practice should be considered harmful until proven safe. Decades of observations and testing should occur before introducing substances to human exposure. The potential harm caused by fluoride in the water, heavy metals in vaccines, aspartame in our foods, and the aftermath of oil spills on aquatic life should be rigorously examined for extended periods of time before declaring such practices safe. And of course the effect of all combinations of such foreign substances must be considered in this experimentation process. Unfortunately the mighty dollar speaks louder than human safety when it comes to these agents, and conventional medicine has clearly dropped the ball in preserving and protecting human health.

Conventional medicine has actually become part of the problem of declining healthcare itself. Not only do traditional providers react to problems once they are present and demand scientific proof; the therapies utilized often impose significant harms. From pharmaceuticals to aggressive surgeries, numerous adverse reactions and bad outcomes can occur.[205] One only needs to listen to television advertisements of pharmaceuticals to appreciate the laundry list of potential harmful effects new drugs may cause. Unfortunately public education and awareness concerning environmental toxins and industry chemicals pale in comparison to drug advertisements. Because pharmaceuticals are "big business" with deep pockets, their ability to influence government agencies, politicians, and providers into using their products is quite strong. No such company or agency focused on prevention exists that can compete with such resources.

Given these progressive developments over the last century, trends demonstrate the failures of conventional medicine in promoting better health and quality of life through an efficient use of limited resources. With Obamacare, efforts to refocus attention toward prevention are being attempted, but honestly the attempts are drops in a very large bucket. Conventional medicine and the American healthcare

---

[205] Centers for Disease Control (CDC). "Adults and older adult adverse drug events." CDC.gov, 2012. Retrieved from http://www.cdc.gov/medicationsafety/adult_adversedrugevents.html.

industry are powerful institutions, and shifting practices toward prevention while financial incentives to increase services and product sales are still in place is nearly impossible to achieve. If changes are to be made, they must start with the individual. Individuals must make the choice to educate themselves about true health practices and to pursue them while supporting alternative solutions.

Rethinking Drugs and Pharmaceuticals

Envisioning a world without medications and drugs is challenging to say the least. The pharmaceutical industry is one of the largest commercial sectors in the world. In fact five of the top ten research and development firms around the globe are pharmaceutical companies. Projections currently for 2016 estimate that the pharmaceutical industry will be worth approximately $1.2 trillion.[206] And while the United States and Europe represent the major markets for medications and drugs, emerging countries are progressively comprising larger market shares, supporting the pervasive nature of this industry.[207] With more and more nations embracing pharmaceutical use, one would expect the advantages of medication management to far outweigh the costs. However, this is often not the case.

Consider the economics of the pharmaceutical situation first. Each year over $135 million is spent on research and development of new drugs. But despite over thirty-two hundred drugs being in the development phase, only thirty-five new drugs were introduced in

---

[206] International Federation of Pharmaceutical Manufacturers and Associations (IFPMA). "The pharmaceutical industry and global health: Facts and figures 2012." IFPMA.org, 2013. Retrieved from http://www.ifpma.org/fileadmin/content/Publication/2013/IFPMA - Facts And Figures 2012 LowResSinglePage.pdf.
[207] Ibid.

2011. Not only does it take an average of four to six years to develop a new drug, but the cost of developing a single new agent is $1.3 billion.[208] It is no wonder pharmacy prices to fill a prescription often prompt a consideration to take out a new personal loan. Of course these figures reflect cutting-edge medications recently developed. Older, established medications and generic drugs are much less in price since greater competition among manufacturers exists. But even these medications often have inflated price tags to compensate for these extreme research and development costs.

From an economic perspective alone, in a healthcare industry with limited resources, the rationale of providing expensive medications to consumers makes little sense. But then again placing a price tag on health and quality of life is difficult. Though healthcare access is far from equitable in the United States, pharmaceutical companies still realize a market will exist for the best treatments available. But are these actually the best approaches to good health? In order to answer this question, examining the costs and benefits of drug therapies and comparing these therapies to alternatives approaches must be performed. In the balance, drugs may not offer the advantages they supposedly claim to provide.

Inherently, problems with medications naturally exist. After all, medications are not natural substances that would be included in our diets, lifestyles, and activities otherwise. Medications require knowledge of prescribing information, possible side effects, possible limitations, and proper administration. According to the World Health Organization, 50 percent of all medications are prescribed, dispensed, or sold inappropriately. And over half of all patients taking

---

[208] Ibid.

medications take them incorrectly.[209] As a result adverse events and outcomes are common when considering pharmaceuticals. Each year in the United States alone, over 700,000 emergency room visits are due to adverse drug reactions, and over 120,000 of these require hospitalizations.[210] Pharmaceuticals are clearly not without some serious concerns.

Medications and pharmaceuticals have dramatically improved health in many ways. But just because some medications offer tremendous benefits does not mean medication therapies should be the primary approach to healthcare in every instance. For example, penicillin offered dramatic benefits to health through the ability to treat a variety of bacterial infections. Today, however, antibiotics seem to be the answer to every sniffle, cough, and sneeze. According to the World Health Organization, 60 percent of all viral upper respiratory tract infections are treated with antibiotic despite having no benefit whatsoever.[211] In fact this overuse of antibiotics has led to increasing degrees of bacterial resistance to treatment. More aggressive infections are thus developing with fewer options of care. In this scenario, drugs are clearly not the answer.

Other problems related to pharmaceuticals involve polypharmacy, where individuals take a plethora of drugs for various health disorders. Just as environmental agencies rarely know the combination of effects of different chemicals, pesticides, and insecticides, the complex interaction among several different medications is typically not known and rarely studied. The question is then raised as to why

---

[209] World Health Organization (WHO). "Medicines: Rational use of medicines." WHO.int, 2010. Retrieved from http://www.who.int/mediacentre/factsheets/fs338/en/.

[210] CDC, 2012.

[211] WHO, 2010.

conventional medicine demands high levels of scientific proof for alternative approaches to health yet prescribes hundreds of drugs that have yet to be tested in combinations. These issues become increasingly important in older individuals whose bodies may be less tolerant of complex drug interactions. Polypharmacy also increases the chance medications will be taken incorrectly. In fact even in the absence of polypharmacy, poor medication compliance and failure to follow instructions are more common than not.

The average person in the United States spends just under eight hundred dollars a year on prescription medications.[212] This does not include over-the-counter medications, which roughly increase annual costs by four hundred dollars per person.[213] Economic costs to individuals and to society reflect significant disadvantages related to the pharmaceutical industry. This combined with antibiotic resistance increases, adverse events, medication errors, polypharmacy, and misuse of medications all serve to undermine the benefit these agents provide in overall health. But perhaps this is the best option available. Or perhaps not.

In evaluating alternatives to medications, a wide spectrum of options exist. Alternative healthcare approaches consist of several different types of strategies including acupuncture, manipulative therapies, stress management, biofeedback, nutritional treatments, and others. In addition to these, other natural efforts involving diet, exercise, and lifestyle change offer preventative measures to avoid illness and

---

[212] Health Care Cost Institute (HCCI). "Spending on prescriptions 2011." *Health Care Cost and Utilization Report: 2011,* 2012. Retrieved from http://www.health-costinstitute.org/files/HCCI_IB4_Prescriptions.pdf.

[213] Consumer Healthcare Products Association (CHPA). "The value of OTC medicine to the United States." CHPA.org, 2012. Retrieved from http://www.chpa.org/ValueofOTCMeds2012.aspx.

disease. Still others address removal of toxins from the body, such as chelation treatments. Thus examining alternatives to medications is challenging due to their broad spectrum of types. Recent studies, however, suggest that such options are increasingly common even in the United States with dollars spent on the alternative healthcare industry in excess of $34 billion a year.[214] Based on this figure alone, a significant number of healthcare consumers in the United States have sought other solutions outside of traditional pharmaceuticals.

In one study examining research from 1999 through 2004, an estimate of cost effectiveness of alternative healthcare therapies was examined in comparison to conventional medicine. Overall, a total of fifty-six studies were analyzed. The authors concluded in specific instances that alternative medicine approaches were more favorable than traditional approaches despite a paucity of research available for review.[215] Examples of these specific instances include acupuncture for migraines, manipulative therapies for neck pain, spa therapy for Parkinsonism, stress management therapy for cancer patients, and a few others. These limited conclusions identified these settings not because other situations were clearly not cost effective but because research supporting other settings had yet to be done.[216] Likewise the study did not address efforts toward health preservation and disease prevention through proactive strategies.

Disadvantages of alternative therapies in comparison to medications are also less significant. Herbal remedies can cause adverse reactions and side effects just as medications can, and polypharmacy

---

[214] Herman, Patricia M., Benjamin M. Craig, and Opher Caspi. "Is complementary and alternative medicine (CAM) cost-effective? A systematic review." *BMC Complementary and Alternative Medicine* 5, no. 1 (2005): 11-40.
[215] Ibid.
[216] Ibid.

and misuse can also occur. However, other alternative approaches that do not utilize chemicals and herbal supplements carry very little risk. Despite common criticisms that manipulative therapies increase risks for spinal injuries, the actual occurrence of such problems is incredibly low. And preventative measures such as eating well, exercising, and avoiding detrimental environments have essentially no potential for harm. The most commonly cited disadvantage of alternatives to medications is their lack of scientific proof. But even this area of weakness (according to conventionalists) is rapidly changing as new studies are increasingly being conducted.

In summary, pharmaceuticals (like conventional medicine) have established a stronghold in many cultures and societies as the primary means by which healthcare is achieved. The increasing appetite for advancing profits continues, resulting in the industry criticizing alternatives while promoting its own costly products. From unethical advertising to skyrocketing prices, the industry has exceeded its ability to provide a real service to health-seeking individuals. Based on costs and benefits, using resources in more productive and less harmful approaches to health seems to make better sense (cents).

A Different Approach to Health

Having discussed the major aspects of conventional medicine and modern pharmaceuticals, the need for alternative ways to approach health is evident. Unlike conventional healthcare, wherein utilization of products and services is driven by the demand for profits, other options of care rely on health measures as their primary incentive. A great example of such an option is anti-aging medicine, which has only recently gained increasing nationwide attention. Rather than approach health through medications, surgeries, and conventional measures, anti-aging specialists focus on nutrition, supplements, exercise, and avoidance of toxins as the primary means to gain health and extend life. And because these choices lack any significant attachment to reimbursement of services, individuals have a wide range of options of care for less cost and greater benefit.

Today fitness gyms are located in every neighborhood, and the importance of a healthy diet has become common knowledge. But in the mid-twentieth century these revelations were underappreciated. Jack Lalanne, the now-famous bodybuilder and health guru, opened the first fitness gym in Oakland, California, in 1936. From that time forward he became the well-known advocate for proper diet and exercise in attaining true health, and the extent to which these messages are now readily accepted can be greatly attributed to him.[217] Interestingly these same messages form the foundation in anti-aging medicine. Prevention of ill health and promotion of good health is far less costly than conventional treatments of disease, and likewise these approaches begin where disease processes might originate rather than focusing on the later effects.

Nutrition and dietary supplements represent a cornerstone of anti-aging healthcare. Proper nutrients, vitamins, and minerals provide the body with necessary tools to promote health and prevent disease. Likewise these efforts are life necessities, unlike medications, which are artificial. One has to eat to survive, so why not choose foods and supplements that also encourage longevity and quality of life? The same cannot be said of medications or of surgeries. Proper nutrition

---

[217] Goldstein, Richard. "Jack Lalanne, founder of modern fitness movement, dies at 96." *New York Times*, 2011. Retrieved from http://www.nytimes.com/2011/01/24/sports/24lalanne.html?_r=0.

provides antioxidants and other agents that boost the immune system, help achieve hormonal balance, and optimize tissue cell functions. In the absence of these substances, the potential for illness is increased, and longevity on average is reduced. Even conventional medicine appreciates this simple fact, but the bulk of its effort is still invested in diagnostics, prescriptions, and reactive treatments once disease is present. The investment of resources into nutritional education, dietary policies, and research on supplements pales in comparison to these profit-generating pursuits.

In addition to proper exercise and diet, anti-aging medicine and health are best served by avoiding specific substances that are either known to cause illness or have yet to be proven safe. In terms of vaccines, many medications, and most environmental chemicals, avoidance of these foreign substances is advantageous since conventional medicine has yet to prove their benefit and lack of harm. Thus preventative measures naturally encourage avoidance strategies first and foremost. After all if exposure to a toxin never occurs then costly treatments are also avoided and health naturally maintained.

Avoidance strategies involve several lifestyle components. Specific foods like grilled and barbecued meats over high heat should be avoided as should processed meats and foods with high omega-6 fats, and high trans-fats. Foods with preservatives and artificial sweeteners or taste-enhancers like aspartame and MSG should be off limits. Drugs should be examined for safety in detail before adding them to a routine or regimen. And avoidance of environmental toxins in the air, water, and soil is similarly important. While food, vitamins, minerals, supplements, and exercise serve to boost natural defenses against an array of toxins and infectious organisms, nothing can replace avoidance of exposure to these items in the first place.

Of course avoidance requires knowledge and awareness, and science as well as traditional medicine has done a relatively poor job in identifying all the potentially harmful toxins currently present in human environments. Therefore, knowledge guiding avoidance strategies can only go so far. In some cases knowledge of the effects of toxins and their presence offers little opportunity to avoid them because many are so ubiquitous in nature. In these situations avoidance strategies must yield to other efforts to rid the body of existing toxins. While the majority of conventional medicine specialists poorly recognize this as an important health strategy, detoxification strategies are imperative in today's world in promoting optimal health and wellness.

Detoxification efforts, including chelation treatments and extreme vitamin regimens, have been utilized for decades. In fact workers exposed to lead poisoning in World War II received chelation treatments to successfully rid their bodies of lead toxins while incidentally also promoting better heart health. Since that time anti-aging health professionals have realized the benefits that various detoxification methods have in protecting human health. Chelation alone has been found to effectively remove a variety of toxic heavy metals from the body, including mercury, arsenic, lead, cadmium, tin, nickel, copper, rubidium, radioactive cesium, barium, titanium, and many others. By adding chelation agents that bind heavy metals and facilitate their elimination from the body and by taking high-dose vitamins that boost the body's detox mechanisms, the body achieves a state of better health, which in turn adds quality years to life.

Of course diet, exercise, vitamins, avoidance techniques, and detoxification therapies are not nearly as profitable for the health profession and health industry as conventional medicine therapies. Instead such interventions are actually frowned upon by traditionalists when compared to more routine approaches to healthcare. Amazingly the very professionals who fail to thoroughly examine the toxic effects of food additives, pesticides, and other environmental chemicals claim that chelation therapies, detox measures, and natural treatments lack objective proof of benefit! If only conventional medicine would turn the mirror on itself and take a good, long look at its unnatural and reactive approach to health then real progress could be made in truly improving health standards, longevity, and quality of life.

In the next chapters a more in-depth look at nutriceuticals, diet, chelation therapies, detoxification treatments, and hormonal replacement methods will be provided. Having established the widespread presence and harmful effects of environmental toxins, we will investigate effective ways to avoid, eliminate, and recover from their exposure. Having experienced such problems and therapies firsthand, I am in a unique position as both patient and healthcare professional to advocate and explain their utility in promoting better health. With a better understanding of these more natural approaches to better health, one will be more able to discern which interventions offer a more rationale choice. Prevention and health promotion offer more effective and far less costly approaches to better health than reactive, conventional medicine and at the same time reduce the exposure to potential causes of health threats.

CHAPTER 10

Food, Diet, and Nutriceuticals

A key component of anti-aging healthcare and the promotion of wellness involves a good dietary strategy. The human body requires the proper fuel in order for the immune system, hormonal system, and other cellular systems to function optimally. This requirement becomes increasingly important when the body is exposed to invisible toxins and environmental threats. Of course some detrimental substances can enter the body through the diet, while others serve to protect the body from illness. Therefore, knowing how to avoid harmful exposures while enhancing health-promoting foods, vitamins, and supplements is essential.

Healthy Dieting Strategy—Foods to Avoid

During the twentieth century major societal changes occurred that affected dieting habits. With industrialization, mass agricultural efforts developed that utilized increasing amounts of chemicals and pesticides to enhance plant production, while hormones and other chemicals were used to augment livestock production. Secondly, growth of food distribution channels encouraged the increased use of food preservatives to allow longer shelf lives. Lastly, advanced commercialism promoted the use of chemicals and changes in food components to provide more appealing (and often more addictive) food tastes. The combination of these effects has served to lower the quality of the diet while exposing individuals to many harmful, health-depleting foods.

Because of this evolution, avoiding foods and food components that are detrimental to health is the first important dietary strategy to adopt. Many of these components have been found to increase the risk of cancer and other illnesses, while others promote premature aging and reduced quality of life. By knowing which substances to avoid and the common foods that contain these detrimental items, better health, wellness, and longevity are much more likely. The following represents the most common substances that one should avoid in maximizing health.

Refined Sugars—From sugar-sweetened beverages to numerous sugary foods, refined sugar is a real threat to good health. The obesity epidemic and rise in diabetes support this fact. In addition refined sugars, because they are rapidly metabolized, cause rapid spikes in blood sugar after consumption, followed by sudden drops. This yo-yo effect stimulates increased food cravings especially for foods high in sugar content. As a result individuals who eat high-sugar-content foods develop addictive tendencies in their diets. In addition diets high in sugar exceed the body's caloric needs. When this occurs sugars are converted to fatty tissue, which leads to a host of other problems including diabetes and obesity.

Because of these health risks foods with refined sugars like pastries, cakes, candies, jellies, dried fruits, sweetened beverages, ice creams, and cereals with added sugar should be avoided as best as possible or minimized significantly. Instead replace these foods with naturally sweet foods like fruits. And in order to avoid pesticide and chemical exposure among these fruits, choose fresh and organic fruits and wash them thoroughly before eating.

Saturated Fats and Trans-Fats—Unlike unsaturated and polyunsaturated fats, saturated fats as well as trans-fats are detrimental to health and longevity. Not only are saturated fats and trans-fats associated with higher levels of cholesterol and triglycerides, but they are also pro-inflammatory agents, which may cause damage to blood vessel walls and other tissues. This can lead to chronic inflammation, autoimmune disorders, allergies, cancers, atherosclerosis, hypertension, and heart disease as well as other metabolic and degenerative diseases.[218] Saturated fats come from animal byproducts like meats, dairy, and eggs, while trans-fats are hydrogenated or partially hydrogenated oils used to preserve foods. Both should be kept to a minimum in the diet (if not completely avoided) in order to prevent these negative health effects.

Omega-6 Fats—Omega-6 fats are polyunsaturated fats; however, these are also pro-inflammatory in nature and can lead to disease and shortened lifespans. In contrast omega-3 fats are anti-inflammatory and reduce disease and tissue injury while augmenting longevity. Ideally the ratio of omega-6 fats to omega-3 fats in the diet should be relatively even, but in Westernized diets this ratio is closer to sixteen

---

[218] Estadella, Débora, Claudia M. da Penha Oller do Nascimento, Lila M. Oyama, Eliane B. Ribeiro, Ana R. Dâmaso, and Aline de Piano. "Lipotoxicity: effects of dietary saturated and transfatty acids." *Mediators of Inflammation* (2013).

to one![219] Thus, the balance is shifted toward a pro-inflammatory state, leading to reduced health and wellness.

Omeg-6 fats are found in vegetable oils like sunflower, corn, soybean, and cottonseed oil, and these oils have increased exponentially in the diet in the last few decades. In order to promote better health, these oils and omega-6 fats in general should be minimized while increasing the amount of omega-3 fats in the diet. Fish like salmon and mackerel have high amounts of omega-3 fats as does flaxseed oil. In addition omega-3 supplements can be taken, which can also to correct an imbalanced ratio. But even if omega-3 fat supplements are used, efforts to avoid omega-6 fats remain important in protecting health.

Nitrites and Preservatives—As mentioned, foods today commonly contain preservatives to prolong shelf life in stores and to allow for extended times of distribution. Nitrates and nitrites are among the better-known preservatives associated with negative health effects. Both of these substances can be converted to nitrosamines, which have been associated with a variety of different cancer types.[220] In addition to these preservatives, several other chemicals including sulfites and sodium benzoate are used to extend food preservation. While these have been associated with migraines, allergies, and other problems, the truth is the actual toxicity from any of these agents has been poorly studied over extended periods of time or in combination with other agents.

---

[219] Gunnars, Kris. "How to optimize your Omega-6 to Omega-3 ratio." Authority Nutrition, 2013. Retrieved from http://authoritynutrition.com/optimize-omega-6-omega-3-ratio/.

[220] N.A. "Avoid nitrates and nitrites in foods." *Healthy Child, Healthy World*, 2013. Retrieved from http://healthychild.org/easy-steps/avoid-nitrates-and-nitrites-in-food/.

Nitrates and nitrites are commonly found in cured or processed meats such as sausages, some hams, hot dogs, and other deli meats. But preservatives are found in many foods other than these. This makes it absolutely essential to read food ingredient labels to assess which chemicals are included within a food item so avoidance can be practiced. It is also noteworthy that celery juice added to some foods (which contains nitrite) is used as a preservative yet allows manufacturers to still make the claim of a food being nitrite or nitrate free.[221]

Artificial Sweeteners and Taste Enhancers—These additives to foods are well known among the public but poorly known for their detrimental health effects. Substances such as aspartame, sucralose, acefultame, aspartic acid, and monosodium glutamate (MSG) are common ingredients in an array of "diet" drinks and processed foods. These substances have been linked to altered neurochemistry, impaired neurodevelopment, neurotoxicity, cancer, liver disease, diffuse inflammation, and impaired immune function.[222] Needless to say these identified effects are likely just the tip of the iceberg since these substances have similarly been poorly investigated before being released into the market. A great example of this is the presumed weight-loss effects of aspartame. Studies are now reporting weight gain being more common among aspartame users than non-aspartame users.[223] Once again reading labels is important to examine

---

[221] Ibid.

[222] Jockers, David. "Artificial sweeteners and flavor enhancers are dangerous." *Natural News*, 2012. Retrieved from http://www.naturalnews.com/035752_artificial_sweeteners_flavor_chemicals.html.

[223] Swithers, Susan E. "Artificial sweeteners produce the counterintuitive effect of inducing metabolic derangements." *Trends in Endocrinology & Metabolism* 24, no. 9 (2013): 431-441.

ingredients in beverages and foods since these agents in particular are used in numerous food products.

Gluten—The increase in the use of flour and wheat over the last century has been astounding. From breads to breadings, batter to beer, to the inclusion of wheat germ in products like toothpaste, wheat seems to find its way into thousands of food products. Gluten, a key component of wheat, has been definitely shown to cause negative health effects in a large number of people. While a small percentage may suffer from a disorder known as celiac disease, caused by a severe immune reaction to gluten, many others have a less severe reaction that can cause more subtle complaints. This latter group of people represents the more common problem associated with gluten. And the vast majority has no idea what the cause of their problems is.

In these instances the immune system can perceive gluten as a foreign substance and attack it as if it were bacteria. The resultant inflammation then spills over to normal tissues, causing inflammation, tissue and cellular damage, and subsequent dysfunction. Problems can include headaches, fatigue, joint and muscle pains, poor memory, imbalance, digestive complaints, rashes, and sleep disturbances. In addition gluten can result in hormonal imbalances, weight problems, and increased susceptibility to other infections. While not everyone has intolerance to gluten, many experts estimate that more than half the population suffers from gluten-related problems.[224] Therefore avoidance of this wheat-based food is encouraged in order to promote optimal health.

---

[224] Petersen, Vikki, and Richard Petersen. *The Gluten Effect.* Sunnyvale, CA: True Health Publishing, 2009.

AGEs—AGE stands for "advanced glycosylated end-products," which essentially describes sugar molecules attaching themselves to various proteins and enzymes. AGEs can develop both within the body and outside the body, and they are associated with inflammation as well as deterioration of cell function. To a great degree AGEs are associated with aging as these glycosylated proteins cause hardening of blood vessel walls, atherosclerosis, reduced cell membrane function, and a marked increase in inflammatory injury over time.[225] Thus, reducing AGEs in the diet is advantageous to slowing the aging process.

Glycosylation of proteins typically occurs with various forms of heat and cooking. Grilling, frying, and roasting of meats and buttered products promote the highest amount of AGEs, while steaming, boiling, and other forms of cooking result in much lesser amounts. Raw, fresh vegetables and fruits of course have little to no AGEs and represent the healthiest choices.

Healthy Dieting Strategy—Nutriceuticals

While avoiding specific foods and food components is an important way to reduce the exposure to toxins and harmful substances in the diet, another strategy involves selecting specific foods and supplements that naturally augment the body's defense mechanisms. Nutriceuticals are substances naturally found in foods and plants that have both nutritional and health-related functions. By choosing such foods in the diet or taking specific nutriceutical supplements, one can help the body recover from toxin exposures and illnesses in an optimal way. In addition nutriceuticals provide the body with

---

[225] Perricone, Nicholas. *Ageless Face, Ageless Mind: Erase Wrinkles and Rejuvenate the Brain*. Random House LLC, 2007.

the best way to stay healthy while slowing down the aging process. Through antioxidant and anti-inflammatory effects, nutriceuticals offer natural solutions in achieving wellness. The following is a list of nutriceuticals that provide preventative strategies toward health and longevity through dietary measures.

Vitamins—Vitamins represent micronutrients essential to the body's wellbeing. Since the body is unable to manufacture these substances, vitamins must be acquired through the diet or through supplements. In relation to health and longevity, some vitamins are more important than others, however. Among the most important vitamins are vitamin C, vitamin A, vitamin E, vitamin D, and B-complex vitamins. Vitamins A, C, and E have well known antioxidant properties and are able to scavenge free radicals and other toxic metabolism byproducts. As a result these vitamins reduce inflammatory injury to cells and tissues while also performing several important metabolic functions. B-complex vitamins (especially vitamins B12, B6, and folate) are involved in preserving proper cell division and neurologic repair systems. As a result these vitamins reduce cell telomere dysfunctions commonly associated with aging. Vitamin D supplementation has also been associated with longer and healthier telomere function (which relates to healthy cell division and repair) and also increases longevity and health.[226]

Certainly all of these vitamins can be gained from the diet by choosing fresh, organic foods rich in these substances; however, in

---

[226] Richards, Byron J. "Nutrition makes anti-aging possible: Secrets of your telomeres." Wellness Resources, 2013. Retrieved from http://www.wellnessresources. com/health/articles/how_nutrition_makes_anti-aging_possible_secrets_of_your_telomeres/.

order to achieve the doses necessary to optimize anti-inflammatory and anti-aging mechanisms, supplements are often necessary. For example, I have routinely benefitted from dosages of vitamin D between 5,000 and 10,000 IU daily as well as doses of vitamin C at 6,000 IU a day. This is in addition to taking between six and ten multivitamin tablets daily. While specific amounts cannot be recommended in a general fashion, suffice it to say that attaining the amounts of vitamins needed to prevent illness and promote wellness likely requires daily supplementation. Discussing individual needs with an anti-aging specialist can help lead one in the right direction in this regard.

Minerals—Like vitamins, minerals are also essential micronutrients that must be attained through the diet. Several minerals are important in reducing inflammation, repairing tissue damage, promoting healthy cellular functions, and improving longevity. Minerals that are considered most important in this regard include magnesium, zinc, and selenium. Each of these has antioxidant properties, reducing inflammatory effects of free radicals and other substances. Specifically, magnesium facilitates DNA replication within cells while also helping heart, brain, musculoskeletal, and immune system functions. Zinc likewise is involved in DNA repair, while selenium has added benefits in reducing cancer risk. Therefore minerals have many advantages in addition to their antioxidant and anti-inflammatory effects.[227]

As with vitamins, minerals are present within many foods. Zinc can be found naturally in oysters and sesame seeds, while selenium is present in barley, codfish, and mushrooms. However, adequate amounts to optimize the health benefits of these substances may be

---

[227] Ibid.

difficult to achieve through diet alone. Personally I supplemented with fifty milligrams of zinc, eight hundred milligrams of magnesium, and four hundred micrograms of selenium daily when I was undergoing detoxification procedures. These amounts helped rid my body of unhealthy substances while augmenting immune, neurologic, and other organ systems. Discussing supplemental amounts for an array of minerals with a prevention specialist can help outline an individual regimen needed for specific purposes.

Omega-3 Fats—As noted earlier, omega-6 fats have increased in Western diets significantly over the last several decades, but omega-3 fats have not. Despite this fact omega-3 fats are essential to good health and must be attained through the diet or through supplements. Natural sources include kale, Brussel sprouts, spinach, and flaxseed as well as fatty fish like salmon and mackerel. The American diet typically has an excess of omega-6 fats while being deficient in omega-3 fats, and for this reason many anti-aging specialists often offer testing of a person's omega-3 to omega-6 ratio to help guide therapy. Dr. Barry Sears, a leader in the field, advocates taking ultra-refined fish oil in order to receive equal amounts of the omega-3 fats EPA and DHA while minimizing exposure to other toxins. For individuals routinely striving to attain good health, twenty-four hundred milligrams of omega-3 fats from equal amounts of EPA and DHA should be taken daily, while those suffering from inflammatory health conditions should take forty-eight hundred milligrams daily.[228] By including this nutriceutical in the diet, one gains protection against heart disease and stroke, while cognitive function is enhanced.

---

[228] Sears, Barry. *The Omega Rx Zone*. New York, NY: HarperCollins, 2009.

Probiotics—These nutriceuticals literally mean "life-promoting" and provide the body with "good" bacteria, which aid in digestive and immune system health. In fact the digestive tract contains nearly three-quarters of the body's immune system. Deficiencies of these beneficial bacterial organisms or an imbalance between disease-causing and health-protecting organisms make the body more susceptible to infection as well as to cancers. Probiotics typically consist of various live organisms including lactobacillus, bifidobacteria, and several others. Natural sources of probiotics can be found in yogurts, cereals, juices, and granola; however, a number of probiotic supplements exist that provide a variety of probiotic organisms to aid better health.[229]

Carotenoids—These nutriceuticals are plant-based chemicals responsible for providing fruits and vegetables with an array of different colors. Examples of carotenoids specifically include beta-carotene, lycopene, zeaxanthin, and astaxanthin. Each of these agents provides powerful antioxidant activity and thus offers significant anti-inflammatory benefits to the body, and most have vitamin A-like activity as well. Astaxanthin, however, has been found to have the most potent antioxidant effects.[230] As a result the risks of inflammatory diseases, cancers, toxic effects, and aging are all reduced by these substances. Natural sources of carotenoids include darkly pigmented vegetables and fruits like carrots, sweet potatoes, spinach, tomatoes, and others. Astaxanthin is found most commonly in wild salmon. Likewise different carotenoids have varying daily dosage amounts that should

[229] Kovacs, Betty. "Probiotics." *MedicineNet*, 2014. Retrieved from http://www.onhealth.com/probiotics/article.htm.

[230] Mercola, Joseph. "Help make your body 62% stronger—Flood it with this inexpensive nutrient." *Mercola.com*, 2011. Retrieved from http://articles.mercola.com/sites/articles/archive/2011/06/15/benefits-of-astaxanthin-to-your-health.aspx.

be taken to maximize health. For example, beta-carotene is routinely taken in amounts between 25,000 and 50,000 IU a day, while astaxanthin can be taken up to ten milligrams a day.[231] Discussion with a health promotion specialist in this regard is encouraged for specific guidance in dosing.

Polyphenols—These nutriceuticals are naturally occurring plant chemicals that come in a variety of categories. Each category shares a basic structural component that is in fact a phenol ring, and all have significant antioxidant activity protecting the body from inflammatory damage. Specific types of polyphenols include flavonoids, anthocyanidins, isoflavones, catechins, and tannins. These plant nutrients are often concentrated in outer structures of fruits and vegetables like the rind, skin, and peel, but they exist in other parts of these foods as well. In order to attain a variety of polyphenols in the diet, including an array of colored fruits and vegetables in your daily meals is important, including foods that are red, blue, purple, orange, and yellow in color. In addition dark and bright colors consistently have higher amounts of antioxidants in general. For example, dark raspberries, brown coffee, black tea, and dark chocolate are known to be high in antioxidant activity. As a result of these substances, better heart health, lipid levels, digestion, and immune function will result while also reducing inflammation and aging processes.[232]

Of note, one polyphenol has received significant attention recently. Resveratrol is a polyphenol naturally found in grapes and cocoa, and

---

[231] Ibid.

[232] Trivieri, Jr., Larry. "Polyphenols: Why to eat plenty of fresh fruits and vegetables." *Integrative Health Review*, 2011. Retrieved from http://www.integrativehealthreview.com/eating-nutrition/polyphenols-why-to-eat-plenty-of-fresh-fruits-and-vegetables/.

many individuals consume this substance while drinking red wine. Resveratrol has been found to not only provide antioxidant activity, but it also speeds energy production and activities within cells while slowing the aging process.[233] Supplements of this compound can be taken in amounts up to five hundred milligrams daily with good effects. Other polyphenols can be acquired through products like apple polyphenol extract and pomegranate flavonoid extract.

Coenzyme Q10—This nutriceutical is actually present in most cellular organisms and is intimately involved in the cellular energy pathway of the body. Without coenzyme Q10, the ability to generate cellular energy would be significantly reduced. But in addition to having energy benefits, coenzyme Q10 is also a powerful antioxidant that enhances immune system function while protecting the brain and other tissues from injury. Coenzyme Q10 is naturally found in meats, poultry, and fish as well as in some vegetables, nuts, and canola oil. Dosage amounts of up to three hundred milligrams a day can be taken to enhance wellness and health.[234]

Amino Acid Supplements—While amino acids are routinely important for building proteins throughout the body, specific amino acids and amino acid combinations have targeted effects in helping promote health and wellness. One such amino acid is theanine, which is a non-dietary amino acid found in green teas. Theanine has been found to protect the body and brain from both physiological and

---

[233] Castillo, Michelle. "Resveratrol does provide anti-aging benefits, study shows." CBS News, 2013. Retrieved from http://www.cbsnews.com/news/resveratrol-does-provide-anti-aging-benefits-study-shows/.

[234] Skae, Teya. "Energy enzyme CoQ10." *Natural News*, 2008. Retrieved from http://www.naturalnews.com/024833_CoQ10_energy_supplement.html.

psychological stress. At the same time theanine enhances cognition and improves concentration.[235] Other amino acid-like nutriceuticals include carnitine and carnosine. Carnitine is composed of two amino acids (lysine and methionine), and it provides antioxidant effects while also facilitating lipid metabolism. As a result it reduces the risk of heart disease, reduces atherosclerosis risk, and protects the body from inflammatory damage.[236] Lastly, carnosine, which is composed of beta-alanine and histidine, is important in preventing and reversing glycosylation of proteins that result in AGEs. In addition to reducing heart-disease risk and reversing atherosclerotic change of blood vessels, carnosine slows the aging process as well. Dosage amounts of carnosine are usually around one thousand milligrams daily, while those of carnitine are five hundred milligrams daily.[237]

Herbal Supplements—Understanding the basics of herbal nutriceuticals can be difficult, but many of these compounds have provided health benefits for centuries, while all of course are natural in origin rather than pharmaceutically developed. Three in particular are noteworthy in terms of health promotion, anti-aging, and disease prevention. These include curcumin, ginkgo biloba, and ashwaganda. Curcumin is an herbal agent known to inhibit a variety of enzymes involved in the body's inflammatory pathways. As a result curcumin regulates the inflammatory process within the body, reducing

---

[235] Kimura, Kenta, Makoto Ozeki, Lekh Raj Juneja, and Hideki Ohira. "L-Theanine reduces psychological and physiological stress responses." *Biological psychology* 74, 1 (2007): 39-45.

[236] Phillip, John. "Super nutrient duo carnosine and carnitine attacks disease." *Natural News*, 2010. Retrieved from http://www.naturalnews.com/030743_carnitine_disease.html.

[237] Ibid.

negative effects resulting from toxins, free radicals, and pro-inflammatory agents.[238] Ginkgo biloba is an ancient herb and well-known antioxidant and substance that enhances tissue utilization of oxygen. Ginkgo has been effectively used to enhance memory and concentration, alleviate depression, improve vision, and improve circulation.[239] Ashwaganda from India has been found to have profound anti-stress effects in addition to anti-inflammatory benefits. Specifically ashwaganda is known to relieve anxiety, increase energy, and improve cognition.[240]

In contrast to medications, surgeries, and other conventional strategies of healthcare, the strategies involving diet and nutrition outlined in this chapter offer natural, proactive measures to attaining health and wellbeing. By avoiding substances known to cause inflammation, to stress the body, and to increase the vulnerability to illness, one can naturally provide the body with a greater capacity to maintain health. By providing nutritional supplements that augment the body's defense systems while reducing inflammatory damage, one can gain greater longevity as well as quality of life. Adopting these habits will greatly improve your health at a fraction of the expense charged by conventional therapies, and unlike traditional therapies these dietary strategies will not introduce new potential toxins into your body.

---

[238] Mercola, Joseph. "Curcumin relieves pain and inflammation for osteoarthritis patients." Mercola.com, 2011. Retrieved from http://articles.mercola.com/sites/articles/archive/2011/01/31/curcumin-relieves-pain-and-inflammation-for-osteo-arthritis-patients.aspx.

[239] N.A. "Ginko biloba." *Herbal Wisdom*, 2010. Retrieved from http://www.herbwis-dom.com/herb-ginkgo-biloba.html.

[240] Singh, Narendra, Mohit Bhalla, Prashanti de Jager, and Marilena Gilca. "An overview on Ashwagandha: A rasayana (rejuvenator) of Ayurveda." *African Journal of Traditional, Complementary and Alternative Medicines* 8, 5S (2011).

CHAPTER 11

Chelation, Detoxification, and Hormonal Replacement

Throughout medical school and my medical residency, not once was chelation or detoxification treatments discussed to any significant degree. One would surmise that such therapies failed to exist or be of any benefit at all, but in actuality quite the reverse is true. Effective chelation therapies have been around since the 1930s, and ample evidence that detoxification effectively improves health exists. It remains a mystery as to why conventional therapies ignore this powerful and effective intervention. Even today (with the exception of California and parts of southern Florida) most of the country remains unaware of these effective health measures. So instead of actually getting to the root cause of the health problem, expensive and potentially toxic new medicines are consumed, which many times only serves to treat the symptoms rather than the actually illness.

In this chapter chelation, detoxification, and hormone replacement therapies will be discussed. These therapies allow the toxins that have built up in the body to be more rapidly and thoroughly removed so health can be restored. Heavy metals, pesticides, herbicides, and a host of other chemicals to which we are exposed every day can gradually accumulate in the body, causing dysfunction of normal bodily systems. Over time this accumulation results in increasing vulnerabilities, leading to illness, poor health, and shortened lifespans. And conventional therapies do little to assist the body in getting rid of these substances. In fact they oftentimes expose the body to additional toxins and harmful agents. Gaining insights into these more effective health strategies can thus offer safer and more effective alternatives in the pursuit of wellness and longevity.

The Basics of Detoxification

In order to appreciate how to actually detoxify the body of harmful chemicals and substances, first an understanding of the body's natural detoxification systems is needed. Detoxification is typically divided into two main phases. Phase one of detoxification involves changing foreign chemicals and unwanted substances into electrically charged compounds. An array of enzymes in the body is responsible for taking these chemicals that are not soluble and transforming them into molecules that have a positive or negative electrical charge. Through oxidation or reduction reactions, oxygen or hydroxyl groups are added to these molecules, which can then be further detoxified by phase two of detoxification.[241] Ultimately this results in the ability of the body to eliminate these toxins, thus restoring better health.

Phase one of detoxification occurs throughout the body in various organ systems, but by far the liver is the most important organ involved in this process. Despite phase one of detoxification utilizing

---

[241] N.A. "Phases of detoxification." *Herbs2000.com*, 2014. Retrieved from http://www.herbs2000.com/h_menu/det_phases.htm.

more than fifty enzymes to modify harmful toxins, the cytochrome p450 enzyme system, which is primarily housed in the liver, accounts for a majority of these reactions. In addition to the liver, the kidney, lungs, muscles, brain, heart, skin, and intestinal tract also have detoxification enzymes, but the vast majority of phase one of detoxification still occurs in the liver itself.[242] Therefore the liver remains the primary organ needed to effectively rid the body of foreign toxins that are introduced from the environment.

Other than proper general nutrition and avoidance of toxins, the ability to augment the enzyme systems involved in phase one of detoxification is mainly accomplished through mineral supplementation. Several minerals are used as cofactors in these enzyme reactions, and therefore including mineral supplements can boost the body's natural detoxification abilities. Zinc, iron, molybdenum, magnesium, selenium, manganese, and sulfur are examples of needed minerals that facilitate these detoxification processes, enabling better elimination of toxins from the body.[243] While many of these can be attained from the diet, as previously noted, being able to maintain consistent levels of these minerals often requires supplements to be taken. In addition the presence of heavy metal toxins in the body often interferes with the function of these enzymes.[244] As will be discussed later, chelation therapies can be important in this situation in removing heavy metals and allowing enzyme function to return to normal.

While phase one of detoxification changes potentially harmful chemicals into electrically charged compounds, phase two of detoxification subsequently converts these compounds into water-soluble

---

[242] Ibid.
[243] Ibid.
[244] Ibid.

forms. This conversion allows these substances to enter the blood-stream and to be eliminated through the urine in most instances. A variety of reactions occurs to accomplish this task. But while this aspect of phase two of detoxification is important, this phase also helps rid the body of many other byproducts left over from phase-one reactions.[245] Oxygen-free radicals and other charged molecules can accumulate after phase-one enzyme activity, causing tissue and cellular damage if not addressed. Phase-two detoxification therefore is not only important in completing the conversion of foreign chemicals into compounds that can be eliminated, but it is similarly important in protecting the body from these other particles.[246]

With this in mind, several antioxidants can be taken that facilitate phase two of detoxification. For example, alpha-lipoic acid (ALA) is a highly reactive antioxidant and free-radical scavenger found in spinach and liver. Consuming ALA in the diet or through supplements not only helps phase two of detoxification but also enhances vitamin B12 activity while boosting the potency of other antioxidant vitamins like vitamin C and vitamin E. In addition, as will be mentioned later, ALA is a natural chelation agent facilitating the removal of some heavy metals.[247] Over the course of several years when I was undergoing detoxification procedures, I routinely took ALA in dosages of eighteen hundred milligrams daily. This in combination with other agents allowed me to eventually regain my health.

Another important antioxidant involved in phase two of detoxification is glutathione. Glutathione is a tri-peptide, meaning it is

---

[245] Ibid.

[246] Ibid.

[247] N.A. "Alpha lipoic acid." *Herbs2000.com*, 2014. Retrieved from http://www.herbs2000.com/h_menu/alpha_lipoic.htm.

composed of three different amino acids (cysteine, glycine, and glutamic acid). Unfortunately the body is unable to absorb glutathione when taken orally, but by taking adequate amounts of these amino acids, one is able to produce glutathione in normal amounts. N-acetyl cysteine (NAC) is therefore often recommended as a supplement to promote higher production of glutathione within the body.[248] Anti-aging specialists recommended six hundred milligrams daily of NAC for this purpose. Methylsulfonyl methane (MSM) is also helpful in increasing the production of glutathione as are vitamins B6 and B12. Like ALA, glutathione is a powerful antioxidant and free-radical scavenger helping rid the body of toxic inflammatory particles often generated by phase-one detoxification and by foreign chemicals themselves.[249] Taking supplements to facilitate its production greatly aids the body in overcoming the effects of environmental toxins.

In addition to ALA, MSM, and NAC, several other agents can be included in the diet to augment antioxidant effects and phase-two detoxification. Some examples include beta-carotene, bioflavonoids, coenzyme Q10, manganese, zinc, selenium, methionine, quercetin, and vitamins A, C, and E. Vitamin C, selenium, and methionine specifically enhance glutathione activity while also providing antioxidant effects independently. In addition to consuming foods that are high in these nutrients, supplementation is often beneficial in further enhancing the body's ability to eliminate toxins.[250] Anti-aging specialists specifically are accustomed to recommending these agents

---

[248] N.A. "Glutathione." *Herbs2000.com*, 2014. Retrieved from http://www.herbs2000.com/amino_acids/glutathione.htm.

[249] Ibid.

[250] Ibid.

and have a working knowledge of the optimal dosages required for this purpose.

The Basics of Chelation

The word "chelation" refers to the ability of a compound to attach itself to another toxic substance and facilitate its removal from the body. Specifically, chelation has come to refer to the removal of heavy metals from the body as a means to promote better health. Despite its relative lack of use in conventional medicine today, chelation has been utilized since World War I, when poison arsenic gases (called lewisite) contaminated soldiers, causing a host of health problems. Dimercaprol was the first chelation agent introduced then, which bound arsenic to its sulfur groups, allowing solubility and elimination.[251] Since that time several other synthetic amino acid compounds have been developed that are more effective at removing heavy metals from the body with fewer side effects. But despite decades of evidence supporting the benefits of chelation therapy in removing mercury, arsenic, lead, iron, plutonium, and uranium from the body, conventional medical organizations continue to ignore these positive effects.

Today both natural and synthetic chelating agents exist that help rid the body of heavy metal toxins. Heavy metals interfere with detoxification enzymes while gradually accumulating in increasing amounts in the body's tissues. Therefore removal of these toxic substances is important especially since exposure to these agents in our environment is rapidly increasing as well. Natural chelating agents in foods should be included in the diet to facilitate the body's normal

---

[251] Dyro, Frances M. "Neurological manifestations of arsenic poisoning." Medscape, 2012. Retrieved from http://emedicine.medscape.com/article/1174215-overview.

detoxification mechanisms while also reducing the need for synthetic chelators. Examples of such foods include citrus fruits like lemons and limes, cilantro, and selenium, which bind mercury; garlic, which binds lead; and chorella, which is a freshwater algae noted to help eliminate mercury.[252]

In addition to these foods and minerals that naturally chelate heavy metals, the body uses a variety of amino acids to serve this purpose as well. Cysteine, histidine, glutathione, methionine, and lysine are amino acids and peptides that chelate heavy metals within cells and thus enhance cellular function. By ensuring an adequate amount of protein exists in the diet, a continuous supply of these amino acids and peptides is provided, allowing optimal natural chelation effects.[253] Supplements NAC and MSM have likewise been described previously in their effects in promoting glutathione production, which notably has both detoxification and chelation effects.

In addition to natural chelation agents, several synthetic compounds are used routinely for chelation therapies. Common agents include DMSA, DMPS, and EDTA, all of which are typically administered through intravenous routes. DMSA has been used since the 1960s and is used to chelate lead, arsenic, and mercury. DMPS, which is an ester of DMSA, was later developed in Russia and is used to chelate mercury as well as cadmium. Lastly EDTA is commonly used to chelate lead from the body in addition to some other less

---

[252] Dunbar, Joseph. "Which natural herbs can be taken for chelation?" *Livestrong.com*, 2013. Retrieved from http://www.livestrong.com/article/199912-what-natural-herbs-can-be-taken-for-chelation/.

[253] Whitaker, Julian, MD. "All about chelation." *NaturalNews.com*, 2009. Retrieved from http://www.naturalnews.com/027338_lead_chelation_health.html.

common heavy metals.[254] In fact EDTA was used first to treat World War II soldiers exposed to lead poisoning and resulted in profound improvements in vision, hearing, memory, and energy in these individuals. Incidentally those treated who had existing heart disease were also noted to have reduced chest pain and improved circulation, thus supporting the more widespread benefits of chelation therapy.[255]

While each of these agents is preferentially provided through the intravenous route, oral and suppository routes are also available. Notably, however, the oral route often allows reduced availability of the chelating agent for effect. I have personally had great success with suppository forms of EDTA in combination with oral forms of DMSA and DMPS. With this combination and the use of natural chelating agents as supplements, I eventually became free of toxic heavy metals over a three-year period. As a result I had increased energy, resolution of depression, and greater fluency of my speech. While detoxification therapies resulted in their own set of benefits, the addition of chelation to eliminate heavy metals from my body furthered my improvement and returned me to a normal state of health.

A Fresh Perspective on Hormonal Therapies

As with detoxification strategies and chelation therapy, the views on hormone replacement therapy (HRT) between conventional medicine specialists and anti-aging specialists are quite different. Since prior studies suggested estrogen replacement therapy in women caused notable increases in breast cancer and heart disease,

[254] Pizzorno, Joseph E., and Michael T. Murray, eds. *Textbook of Natural Medicine.* New York, NY: Elsevier Health Sciences, 2012.
[255] Whitaker, 2009.

the traditional medical community has taken a hard stance against HRT in many postmenopausal women. Likewise advertisements by lawsuit-happy attorneys today highlight mainstream views against testosterone replacement in men, claiming numerous bad outcomes in men receiving these therapies. But despite these perspectives the fact of the matter remains that hormonal replacement has distinct advantages to health as we age. The lack of appreciation of this fact among conventional medicine providers often stems from a degree of ignorance about the details of prior studies and about the specific therapies themselves.

From a personal perspective, a family member who recently underwent a hysterectomy was told progesterone replacement was completely unnecessary as part of her ongoing care after surgery. Progesterone in essence is a hormone that opposes estrogen, resulting in a balance that fosters optimal wellness. Progesterone, which naturally begins to decline after thirty-five years of age, dramatically falls after removal of the ovaries. In addition to its ability to prevent estrogen excess, progesterone also reduces heart-disease risk, enhances the ability to sleep, deters depression and mood swings, and exerts an anti-proliferative effect, reducing the risk of breast cancer and leukemia. The shortsighted view that progesterone replacement is not needed post-hysterectomy neglects to consider all of these health benefits HRT provides.

For women, two key hormones to be considered with aging involve estrogen and progesterone, which exist in a balance to promote optimal wellbeing. However, over time, both levels tend to fall as ovarian production declines. Deficiencies of progesterone have been mentioned already, but estrogen deficiency causes additional problems, including excessive wrinkling of the skin, bone loss, memory decline, mood swings, and hot flashes.[256] Low estrogen levels are also associated with increased LDL cholesterol levels and lower HDL levels, which serve to advance atherosclerosis.[257] Thus replacement of both of these hormones becomes increasingly important with age as a means to preserve cardiovascular function, reduce cancer risk, maintain bone and muscular health, and enhance quality of life.

In addition to declines of estrogen and progesterone in women as a result of aging, environmental factors are also important. Estrogen dominance, which describes an imbalance of estrogen in relation to progesterone, is often triggered from external exposure to other substances. Pesticides, herbicides, polychlorinated biphenols, and other chemicals can expose the body to substances that are converted to estrogens. Likewise obesity and excess caloric intake common in Westernized diets and cultures also increase estrogen production in the body.[258] As increased estrogen develops in relation to progesterone, estrogen dominance develops, resulting in a variety of symptoms. These may include breast tenderness, cystic disease, anxiety, and fibroids as well as weight gain. Other common complaints also include depression, reduced energy, and migraines.[259]

Male-specific hormones primary involve testosterone, although, as with women, hormonal ratios are important. The ratio of testosterone to estrogen, for example, significantly changes over time with young men averaging ratios of fifty to one, while middle-aged and

[256] N.A. "Female hormone restoration." *Life Extension Foundation*, 2014. Retrieved from http://www.lef.org/protocols/female_reproductive/female_hormone_restoration_01.htm.

[257] Ibid.

[258] Giampapa, Vincent C. *The Principles and Practice of Anti-aging Medicine for the Clinical Physician*. Denmark: River Publishers, 2012.

[259] Ibid.

older men have ratios of twenty to one and eight to one respectively. This natural decline in testosterone, however, is associated with several health complaints, including reduced libido, reduced energy, depression, and weight gain. Likewise lower testosterone levels result in bone and muscle loss, anemia, indecisiveness, and loss of memory.[260] In addition, low testosterone levels are associated with elevated cancer risk and prostate gland enlargement.[261] But despite this evidence critics of testosterone replacement abound.

One of the important aspects of HRT from an anti-aging specialist's view is to use bio-identical forms of hormones when replacing specific hormone substances. The studies that have suggested detrimental effects from HRT have utilized synthetic hormone chemicals, which significantly differ from human hormones. Bio-identical hormones, however, which are plant based, are the same as human hormone structures and have not been associated with these same detrimental effects. In fact bio-identical hormones have been found to have the exact opposite effect in many cases, significantly enhancing overall wellness.[262]

Anti-aging specialists also take a much more gradual and natural approach to HRT compared to conventional medicine providers. Instead of simply adding hormonal medications to symptom complaints, anti-aging specialists measure specific hormone levels over several months to attain an accurate measure of hormonal function. Subsequently if these levels are low, precursors to hormones are given (which are more natural and safer) to assess if the body has a functional reserve to produce hormones itself in a natural way. Only after

---

[260] Ibid.

[261] Ibid.

[262] Ibid.

these measures are performed will the administration of bio-identical HRT be considered.[263] Such an approach is not only more natural but also more cautious overall.

Other natural hormones are also integral to HRT considerations in treating health and wellness. These may include replacement of thyroid hormone, growth factor, melatonin, and even cortisol. However, the ability to detail these specific approaches is beyond the scope of this book. Regardless, the body's hormonal system is critically important in keeping the body in balance, detoxifying substances acquired from the environment, and facilitating quality of life and longevity. By aligning HRT practices with natural replacement hormones and by guiding therapies based on accurate and repetitive measurements, these health-related goals can be readily attained.

For most people who seek medical care, the opportunity to learn about detoxification treatments and chelation therapies is rarely enjoyed. And the discussion concerning hormonal replacement therapy is often centered on inaccurate information and a knee-jerk reaction to options of care. This practice is extremely unfortunate given the potential these treatments have in helping the body eliminate toxins and restoring a healthy balance. The approach taken by most anti-aging specialists is remarkably different in these areas, and time and time again these interventions have been shown to increase lifespan, quality of life, and overall wellbeing. In today's world the exposure to toxins and heavy metals is pervasive, and the human body has limited capacity to deal with such challenges. This ability is compromised even further when dietary inadequacies exist and hormonal imbalances develop. The key to overcoming these difficulties lies within

---

[263] Ibid.

specific treatments that target the underlying issues, and the ones described in this chapter clearly take this approach. Getting to the root of the problem rather than temporarily appeasing symptoms will continue to be the best way of preserving health and the one anti-aging specialists will wholeheartedly embrace.

CHAPTER 12

Conclusion: The Big Picture

For the most part the average life expectancy of Americans has slowly increased over the last century. Even in the last two decades the average life expectancy for men has increased about four years, while women on average live more than two years longer. But these averages neglect to detail the real truth about longevity and quality of life. In many segments of the population, particularly women, the lifespan is shrinking. And when compared to other countries, the United States has fallen from a ranking of twentieth in 1987 to a ranking of thirty-seventh in 2007.[264] Those invested in conventional medicine claim the overall trend supports the rationale of traditional American healthcare. But in reality most of the advances in lifespan have resulted from preventative measures like cessation of smoking.

From the discussions in this book, the real trends in healthcare and in the nation's overall health should be clearer. The US healthcare system is founded upon the same cultural and political foundations as its economic and consumer-based systems. Capitalism has been

---

[264] Patrick, Martin. "Life expectancy declining in many parts of U.S." *World Socialist Web Site*, 2011. Retrieved from http://www.wsws.org/en/articles/2011/06/life-j16.html.

present since its development, and over the course of the last century entrepreneurs, industries, educational systems, politicians, and government have combined to establish a massive, profit-based system that thrives on its progressive utilization by the public. Because of this, reactive healthcare has overtaken preventative efforts, and symptoms are addressed through profit-generating products and services, while root causes are ignored. As a result consumers have come to expect quick fixes instead of self-motivated lifestyle changes. And innovative technologies and drugs are heralded as breakthroughs, while overall health statistically declines.

If these conventional approaches to healthcare were not detrimental enough, similar pressures on health from the environment in which we live have also increased. The food we eat, the water we drink, and the air we breathe now expose us over a lifetime to thousands if not millions of chemicals and synthetic substances that have yet to be proven safe. Safety research fails to consider additive and multiplicative effects that various chemicals may have in combination on health, and the length of evaluation of most research protocols is ridiculously brief in comparison to chemical half-lives. Yet while these safety issues are ignored, the same industries demand extensive verification of the safety and benefit of preventative therapies that compete with conventional medicine ones. The hypocrisy behind such actions only serves to again highlight the need for our current healthcare system and other industries to consistently drive profits upward.

If we are to make a change, the change will have to come from within. Politicians, CEOs, conventional healthcare providers, and other traditional leaders of healthcare are unlikely to make sweeping changes because incentives are stacked against them. And even among the few who may challenge the status quo, the degree of power to change healthcare in a new direction pales in comparison to the power of these massive industries. Change therefore must come from individuals who understand the problem and choose to take a new approach to healthcare. Instead of feeding the existing healthcare machine for minimal returns on investment, individuals will need to educate themselves and pursue a preventative approach to health and wellness. Through a collective voice, policies regarding the environment may change, and through individual health efforts, quality of life and longevity can be enjoyed.

With this perspective in mind, efforts to improve health fall into two main categories. First, the avoidance of toxins, chemicals, vaccinations, electromagnetic radiation, and pollutants offers a major line of defense. Anti-aging specialists have appreciated for years the benefits of minimizing exposure to these harmful substances, and with the number of these agents progressively increasing in the environment, in our food supplies, and among routine healthcare practices, avoidance has become a more important strategy for wellness. Secondly, lifestyles and activities should be adopted that not only promote health but also help the body fight such detrimental substances. Nutriceuticals, organic fruits and vegetables, adequate sleep, exercise, chelation therapies, detoxification methods, and hormone replacement represent the most common strategies in this regard. Interestingly, conventional healthcare places little to no emphasis on these two measures of care despite proven evidence that such methods are effective, less costly, and more natural overall.

Understandably the information provided in this book only scratches the surface in terms of shedding light on major problems with today's current approach to healthcare. Likewise the alternative approaches to health described only serve as a foundation in changing toward a more preventative approach to wellness. However, this knowledge is important in helping to make the decision to change and to appreciate the shortcomings of our current healthcare and environmental policies. The next step thus involves taking this knowledge and pursuing that change with the guidance of anti-aging specialists or other preventative health providers. These specialists view health from a more natural perspective and offer specific as well as thoughtful guidance in how such changes can be made.

The power and predominance of conventional healthcare in today's society are undoubtedly impressive considering that its origins date back only a century and a half. For millennia, herbal and natural therapies have provided advancing health to mankind while at the same time respecting the environment. But while conventional therapies have provided significant breakthroughs in fighting disease in many instances, the detriments they now impose on human health and our environment are substantial. Adequate resources do not exist to continue to fuel this consumption-driven industry, and ultimately healthcare will suffer as a result. These changes are already occurring as those with resources receive better care than those without. Fortunately prevention is available to all, and avoidance, diet, nutrients, and other strategies have much greater long-term benefits on health than those offered by conventional care today. Making the choice to change directions and pursue this approach to wellness allows individuals to reclaim the power needed to truly enjoy healthier lives.

WORKS CITED

ACGME. "2010 ACGME Residency Common Program Requirements." *AMA-ASSN.org*, 2010. http://www.ama-assn.org/resources/doc/rfs/dutyhours.pdf.

Adams, Mike. "Merck vaccine scientist Dr. Maurice Hilleman admitted presence of SV40, AIDS and cancer viruses in vaccines." *Natural News*. Sept. 15, 2011. http://www.naturalnews.com/033584_Dr_Maurice_Hilleman_SV40.html.

Adams, Mike. "What's really in vaccines? Proof of MSG, formaldehyde, aluminum and mercury." *Natural News*. October 24, 2012. http://www.naturalnews.com/037653_vaccine_additives_thimerosal_formaldehyde.html.

Alavanja, Michael C.R., Jane A. Hoppin, and Freya Kamel. "Health Effects of Chronic Pesticide Exposure: Cancer and Neurotoxicity* 3." *Annual. Rev. Public Health* 25 (2004): 155-197.

AlDabal, Laila, and Ahmed S. BaHammam. "Metabolic, endocrine, and immune consequences of sleep deprivation." *The Open Respiratory Medicine Journal* 5 (2011): 31-43.

"Alpha lipoic acid." *Herbs2000.com*, 2014. http://www.herbs2000.com/h_menu/alpha_lipoic.htm.

American Association for Justice. "Preventable medical errors—The sixth biggest killer in America." Justice.org, 2014. http://www.justice.org/cps/rde/justice/hs.xsl/8677.htm.

American Academy of Pediatrics. "Vaccine safety: Examine the evidence." *AAP.Org*. April 2013. http://www2.aap.org/immunization/families/faq/vaccinestudies.pdf.

Auerbach, David I., and Arthur L. Kellermann. "A decade of health care cost growth has wiped out real income gains for an average US family." *Health Affairs* 30, no. 9 (2011): 1630-1636.

"Avoid nitrates and nitrites in foods." *Healthy Child, Healthy World*, 2013. http://healthychild.org/easy-steps/avoid-nitrates-and-nitrites-in-food/.

Beasley, David. "Survey shows more U.S. children getting vaccines." Reuters. Sept. 1, 2011. http://www.reuters.com/article/2011/09/01/usa-vaccines-idUSN1E7801L020110901.

Bidleman, Terry F., Lisa M. M. Jantunen, Paul A. Helm, Eva Brorström-Lundén, and Sirkka Juntto. "Chlordane enantiomers and temporal trends of chlordane isomers in Arctic air." *Environmental Science & Technology* 36, no. 4 (2002): 539-544.

Bienkowski, Brian. "New report: Unregulated contaminants common in drinking water." *Environmental Health News*, 2013. http://www.environmentalhealthnews.org/ehs/news/2013/unregulated-water-contaminants.

Brody, Jane E. "Too many pills for aging patients." *The New York Times*, April 16, 2012. http://well.blogs.nytimes.com/2012/04/16/too-many-pills-for-aging-patients/?_r=0.

Brown, E. Richard. *Rockefeller Medicine Men: Medicine and Capitalism in America*. Los Angeles, CA: University of California Press, 1979.

Brumfield, Ben. "Shift workers beware: Sleep loss may cause brain damage, new research says." CNN.com, 2014. http://www.cnn.com/2014/03/19/health/sleep-loss-brain-damage/.

Cantwell, Alan. "The gay experiment that started AIDS in America." Rense.com. Nov. 27, 2005. http://www.rense.com/general68/gayex.htm.

Castillo, Michelle. "Resveratrol does provide anti-aging benefits, study shows." CBS News, 2013. http://www.cbsnews.com/news/resveratrol-does-provide-anti-aging-benefits-study-shows/.

Centers for Disease Control (CDC). "Adults and older adult adverse drug events." CDC.gov, 2012. http://www.cdc.gov/medicationsafety/adult_adversedrugevents.html.

Centers for Disease Control (CDC). "Medication Safety Basics." CDC.gov. http://www.cdc.gov/medicationsafety/basics.html.

Centers for Medicare and Medicaid Services (CMS). "National health expenditures 2012 highlights." CMS.gov, 2013. http://www.cms.gov/Research-Statistics-Data-and-Systems/Statistics-Trends-and-Reports/NationalHealthExpendData/downloads/highlights.pdf.

Chemicals, U.N.E.P. "Ridding the world of POPs: A guide to the Stockholm Convention on Persistent Organic Pollutants, the Secretariat of the Stockholm Convention and UNEP's Information Unit for Conventions." 2005.

Consumer Healthcare Products Association (CHPA). "The value of OTC medicine to the United States." CHPA.org, 2012. http://www.chpa.org/ ValueofOTCMeds2012.aspx.

De Flora, Silvio, Alberto Quaglia, Carlo Bennicelli, and Marina Vercelli. "The epidemiological revolution of the 20th century." *The FASEB journal* 19, no. 8 (2005): 892-897.

Dellorto, Danielle. "'Dirty Dozen' carries more pesticide residue, group says." CNN.Com, 2010. http://www.cnn.com/2010/HEALTH/06/01/dirty.dozen. produce.pesticide/.

Dunbar, Joseph. "Which natural herbs can be taken for chelation?" Livestrong.com, 2013. http://www.livestrong.com/article/199912-what-natural-herbs-can-be-taken-for-chelation/.

Dyro, Frances M. "Neurological manifestations of arsenic poisoning." Medscape, 2012. http://emedicine.medscape.com/article/1174215-overview.

Ecobichon, Donald J., and Robert M. Joy. *Pesticides and neurological diseases.* Boca Raton, FL: CRC Press, 1993.

"Energy drinks linked to adverse health effects." CNBC.com, 2013. http://www. cnbc.com/id/100581965.

EPA. "Buildings and their impact on the environment: A statistical summary." *Environmental Protection Agency Green Building,* 2009. http://www.epa.gov/ greenbuilding/pubs/gbstats.pdf.

EPA. "Pesticides and Public Health." 2008. http://www.epa.gov/pesticides/health/ public.htm#regulation.

Estadella, Débora, Claudia M. da Penha Oller do Nascimento, Lila M. Oyama, Eliane B. Ribeiro, Ana R. Dâmaso, and Aline de Piano. "Lipotoxicity: effects of dietary saturated and transfatty acids." *Mediators of Inflammation,* 2013.

European Lung Foundation. "Outdoor air pollution: Air quality and health." EuropeanLungFoundation.org, n.d. http://www.european-lung-foundation. org/126-european-lung-foundation-elf-outdoor-air-pollution.htm.

"Female hormone restoration." Life Extension Foundation, 2014. http://www.lef. org/protocols/female_reproductive/female_hormone_restoration_01.htm.

Foster, Susan D. "WHO knew about harm from electromagnetic radiation." InfoWars.com, 2014. http://www.infowars.com/who-knew-about-harm-from-electromagnetic-radiation/.

Gaille, Brandon. "26 energy drink industry statistics and trends." BrandonGaille. com, 2013. http://brandongaille.com/26-energy-drink-industry-statistics-and-trends/.

Gates, Bill. "Innovating to zero." TED, 2010. http://www.ted.com/talks/bill_gates/transcript.

Gervais, Roger R. "Understanding the vaccine controversy." *Nature Life Magazine*, 1996. http://www.naturallifemagazine.com/naturalparenting/vaccines.htm.

Giampapa, Vincent C. *The Principles and Practice of Anti-aging Medicine for the Clinical Physician*. Denmark: River Publishers, 2012.

Gilbert, Beth. "The health risks of energy drinks." *Huffington Post*, 2012. http://www. huffingtonpost.com/2012/10/25/health-risks-energy-drinks_n_2009529. html.

"Ginko biloba." *Herbal Wisdom*, 2010. http://www.herbwisdom.com/herb-ginkgo-biloba.html.

"Global mobile statistics 2014 Part A: Mobile subscribers; handset market share; mobile operators." MobiThinking.com, 2014. http://mobithinking.com/mobile-marketing-tools/latest-mobile-stats/a.

"Glutathione." Herbs2000.com, 2014. http://www.herbs2000.com/amino_acids/glutathione.htm.

GMO Awareness. "GMO risks." GM-Awareness.com, 2011. http://gmo-awareness. com/all-about-gmos/gmo-risks/.

Goldman, G. S., and N. Z. Miller. "Relative trends in hospitalizations and mortality among infants by the number of vaccine doses and age, based on the Vaccine Adverse Event Reporting System (VAERS), 1990–2010." *Human & Experimental Toxicology* 31, no. 10 (2012): 1012-1021.

Goldstein, Richard. "Jack Lalanne, founder of modern fitness movement, dies at 96." *New York Times*, 2011. http://www.nytimes.com/2011/01/24/sports/24lalanne. html?_r=0.

Greene, Deborah. "EMF radiation dangers and protection." YourEnergyMatters. com, 2011. http://debragreene.com/radiation.asp.

Greenguard Certification. "Indoor air quality: Chemicals." Greenguard.org, 2014. http://www.greenguard.org/en/indoorAirQuality/iaq_chemicals.aspx.

Gunnars, Kris. "How to optimize your Omega-6 to Omega-3 ratio." Authority Nutrition, 2013. http://authoritynutrition.com/optimize-omega-6-omega-3-ratio/.

Hagas, Mavda. "BRAG antenna ranking of schools." Electromagnetichealth.org, 2010. http://electromagnetichealth.org/wp-content/uploads/2010/04/BRAG_Schools.pdf.

Hakim, F., Wang, Y., Zhang, S.X., Zheng, J., Yolcu, E.S., Carreras, A., Khalyfa, A., Shirwan, H., Almendros, I., and Gozal, D. "Fragmented sleep accelerates tumor growth and progression through recruitment of tumor-associated macrophages and TLR4 signaling." *Cancer Research*, 2014.

Harvey, Matt. "No, you can't drink…water." The Fix, 2013. http://www.thefix.com/content/water-supply-contamination-trace-pharmaceuticals8666.

Health Care Cost Institute (HCCI). "Spending on prescriptions 2011." *Health Care Cost and Utilization Report: 2011*, 2012. http://www.healthcostinstitute.org/files/HCCI_IB4_Prescriptions.pdf.

"Healthcare statistics in the United States." HealthPAC Online. http://www.healthpaconline.net/health-care-statistics-in-the-united-states.htm.

Herman, Patricia M., Benjamin M. Craig, and Opher Caspi. "Is complementary and alternative medicine (CAM) cost-effective? A systematic review." *BMC Complementary and Alternative Medicine* 5, no. 1 (2005): 11-40.

Horowitz, Leonard G. *Emerging Viruses: AIDS, Ebola & Vaccinations*. Tetrahedron, 1997.

"Immunization schedules." Centers for Disease Control. Jan. 31, 2014. http://www.cdc.gov/vaccines/schedules/.

Information Liberation. "The fluoride conspiracy." 2006. http://www.informationliberation.com/?id=14949.

International Federation of Pharmaceutical Manufacturers and Associations (IFPMA). "The pharmaceutical industry and global health: Facts and figures 2012." IFPMA.org, 2013. http://www.ifpma.org/fileadmin/content/Publication/2013/IFPMA_-_Facts_And_Figures_2012_LowResSinglePage.pdf.

Jaslow, Ryan. "Autism rates rise 30 percent in two-year span: CDC." CBS News, 2014. http://www.cbsnews.com/news/autism-rates-rise-30-percent-in-two-year-span-cdc/.

Jockers, David. "Artificial sweeteners and flavor enhancers are dangerous." *Natural News*, 2012. http://www.naturalnews.com/035752_artificial_sweeteners_flavor_chemicals.html.

Kenny, Tim. "Breastfeeding." *Patient.co.uk*. July 7, 2013. http://www.patient.co.uk/health/breast-feeding.

Kimura, Kenta, Makoto Ozeki, Lekh Raj Juneja, and Hideki Ohira. "L-Theanine reduces psychological and physiological stress responses." *Biological Psychology* 74, 1 (2007): 39-45.

Kovacs, Betty. "Probiotics." *MedicineNet*, 2014. http://www.onhealth.com/probiotics/article.htm.

Lawlis, G. Frank. "The Sleep Solution Workbook." DrPhil.com, n.d. http://www.drphil.com/assets/c/c0f3ab7356c5913f1a91dc7c7c347ecc.pdf.

Leoni, Edgar. *Nostradamus and His Prophecies*. Mineola, NY: Dover Publications Inc., 2000.

Levitt, B. Blake, and Henry Lai. "Biological effects from exposure to electromagnetic radiation emitted by cell tower base stations and other antenna arrays." *Environmental Reviews* 18, no. NA (2010): 369-395.

Lipman, Frank. "13 ways to protect yourself from electromagnetic radiation." DrFrankLipman.com, 2013. http://www.drfranklipman.com/13-ways-to-protect-yourself-from-electromagnetic-radiation/.

Lopez, Alan D. "Morbidity and mortality, changing patterns in the twentieth century." *Encyclopedia of biostatistics* (1998).

Lundy, Karen Saucier, and Sharyn Janes. *Community Health Nursing: Caring for the public's health*. New York, NY: Jones & Bartlett Learning, 2009.

Lutz, Wolfgang, and K. C. Samir. "Global human capital: Integrating education and population." *Science* 333, 6042 (2011): 587-592.

Mackey, Maureen. "Sleepless in America: A $32.4 billion business." *The Fiscal Times*, 2012. http://www.thefiscaltimes.com/Articles/2012/07/23/Sleepless-in-America-A-32-4-Billion-Business?page=0%2C0.

Mann, Denise. "Coping with excessive sleepiness." WebMD, 2010. http://www.webmd.com/sleep-disorders/excessive-sleepiness-10/immune-system-lack-of-sleep.

Mercola, Joseph. "Aspartame: By far the most dangerous substance added to most foods today." Mercola.com, 2011. http://articles.mercola.com/sites/articles/archive/2011/11/06/aspartame-most-dangerous-substance-added-to-food.aspx.

Mercola, Joseph. "Blood on Their Hands: The World's Slickest Con Job and a Stack of Deadly LIES..." Mercola.com, 2010. http://articles.mercola.com/sites/articles/archive/2010/11/04/big-profits-linked-to-vaccine-mandates.aspx.

Mercola, Joseph. "Curcumin relieves pain and inflammation for osteoarthritis patients." Mercola.com, 2011. http://articles.mercola.com/sites/articles/archive/2011/01/31/curcumin-relieves-pain-and-inflammation-for-osteoarthritis-patients.aspx.

Mercola, Joseph. "Help make your body 62% stronger—Flood it with this inexpensive nutrient." Mercola.com, 2011. http://articles.mercola.com/sites/articles/archive/2011/06/15/benefits-of-astaxanthin-to-your-health.aspx.

Mercola, Joseph. "7,000 clinical studies concur—This meat is a clear invitation to cancer..." Mercola.com, 2011. http://articles.mercola.com/sites/articles/archive/2011/04/11/when-are-hotdogs-better-for-you-than-chicken.aspx.

Michigan Department of Community Health. "PBBs (Polybrominated Biphenyls) in Michigan." MDCH, 2011. http://www.michigan.gov/documents/mdch_PBB_FAQ_92051_7.pdf.

Milham, S., and E. M. Ossiander. "Historical evidence that residential electrification caused the emergence of the childhood leukemia peak." *Medical Hypotheses* 56, no. 3 (2001): 290-295.

Miller, G. Tyler Jr., and Scott E. Spoolman. *Sustaining the Earth*. Belmont, CA: Brooks/Cole Cengage Learning, 2010.

Moritz, Andreas. *Vaccine-Nation: Poisoning the Population, One Shot at a Time*. Ener-Chi Wellness Center, 2011.

National Cancer Institute. "Formaldehyde and cancer risk." National Cancer Institute, 2012. http://www.cancer.gov/cancertopics/factsheet/Risk/formaldehyde.

National Safety Council. "Sick building syndrome." National Safety Council, 2009. http://www.nsc.org/news_resources/Resources/Documents/Sick_Building_Syndrome.pdf.

Natural Revolution. "The good, bad and ugly about GMOs." NaturalRevolution.org, 2013. http://naturalrevolution.org/gmo-resources/the-good-bad-and-ugly-about-gmos/.

Natural Standard. "Hormones and antibiotics in food supply." Health24.Com, 2011. http://www.health24.com/Lifestyle/Environmental-health/21st-century-life/Hormones-and-antibiotics-in-food-supply-20130311.

Neustaedter, Randall. "What are the alternatives to vaccinations?" HealthyChild. com. http://www.healthychild.com/what-are-the-alternatives-to-vaccination/.

PANNA. "Pesticides on food." Pesticide Action Network North America, n.d. http://www.panna.org/issues/food-agriculture/pesticides-on-food.

Patrick, Martin. "Life expectancy declining in many parts of U.S." World Socialist Web Site, 2011. http://www.wsws.org/en/articles/2011/06/life-j16.html.

Peltier, Karen. "Volatile Organic Compounds (VOCs): What they're all about." About.com. http://greencleaning.about.com/od/GreenCleaningResources/g/Volatile-Organic-Compounds-Vocs-What-They-Re-All-About.htm.

Perlingieri, Ilya Sandra. "Chemtrails: The consequences of toxic metals and chemical aerosols on human health." GlobalResearch.org, 2014. http://www.globalresearch.ca/chemtrails-the-consequences-of-toxic-metals-and-chemical-aerosols-on-human-health/19047.

Perlmutter, David. *Grain Brain*. New York, NY: Little, Brown & Co., 2009.

Perricone, Nicholas. *Ageless Face, Ageless Mind: Erase Wrinkles and Rejuvenate the Brain*. Random House LLC, 2007.

Petersen, Vikki, and Richard Petersen. *The Gluten Effect*. Sunnyvale, CA: True Health Publishing, 2009.

Petersen, Vikki, and Richard Peterson. *The Gluten Effect*. True Health Publishing, 2009.

"Phases of detoxification." Herbs2000.com, 2014. http://www.herbs2000.com/h_menu/det_phases.htm.

Phillip, John. "Super nutrient duo carnosine and carnitine attacks disease." Natural News, 2010. http://www.naturalnews.com/030743_carnitine_disease.html.

Pimentel, David, Herbert Acquay, Michael Biltonen, P. Rice, M. Silva, J. Nelson, V. Lipner, S. Giordano, A. Horowitz, and M. D'amore. "Environmental and economic costs of pesticide use." *BioScience* 42, no. 10 (1992): 750-760.

Pizzorno, Joseph E., and Michael T. Murray, eds. *Textbook of Natural Medicine*. New York, NY: Elsevier Health Sciences, 2012.

Plinio, Prioreschi. *A History of Medicine: Primitive and Ancient Medicine*. Omaha, NE: Horatius Press, 1995.

Prate, Dawn. "The great thimerosal cover-up: Mercury, vaccines, autism and your child's health." Natural News. Sept. 22, 2005. http://www.naturalnews.com/011764_thimerosal_mercury.html.

Rees, Camilla. "Biological effects of electromagnetic fields." *International Institute for Building-Biology & Ecology: Healthy Bodies Healthy Buildings Conference 2012.* http://www.youtube.com/watch?v=Z88glpsehQY.

Richards, Byron J. "Nutrition makes anti-aging possible: Secrets of your telomeres." Wellness Resources, 2013. http://www.wellnessresources.com/health/articles/how_nutrition_makes_anti-aging_possible_secrets_of_your_telomeres/.

Riedel, Stefan. "Edward Jenner and the history of smallpox and vaccination." *Proceedings (Baylor University Medical Center).* Jan. 2005; 18(1): 21-25.

Safer Chemicals. "Perfluorinated compounds." SaferChemical.org. http://www.saferchemicals.org/resources/chemicals/pfc.html.

Saliba, Andrea. "The poison in our food." *The McGill Daily*, 2014. http://www.mcgilldaily.com/2014/01/the-poison-in-our-food/.

Sanborn, M., K. J. Kerr, L. H. Sanin, D. C. Cole, K. L. Bassil, and C. Vakil. "Non-cancer health effects of pesticides: Systematic review and implications for family doctors." *Canadian Family Physician* 53, no. 10 (2007): 1712-1720.

Sears, Barry. *The Omega Rx Zone.* New York, NY: HarperCollins, 2009.

Sears, Robert W. *The vaccine book: Making the right decision for your child.* Hachette Digital, Inc., 2011.

Segell, Michael. "Is dirty electricity making you sick?" *Prevention*, 2011. http://www.prevention.com/health/healthy-living/electromagnetic-fields-and-your-health.

Singh, Narendra, Mohit Bhalla, Prashanti de Jager, and Marilena Gilca. "An overview on Ashwagandha: A rasayana (rejuvenator) of Ayurveda." *African Journal of Traditional, Complementary and Alternative Medicines* 8, 5S (2011).

Skae, Teya. "Energy enzyme CoQ10." Natural News, 2008. http://www.naturalnews.com/024833_CoQ10_energy_supplement.html.

Smoley, Richard. *The Essential Nostradamus.* New York, NY: Penguin, 2006.

Stellman, Jeanne Mager, Steven D. Stellman, Richard Christian, Tracy Weber, and Carrie Tomasallo. "The extent and patterns of usage of Agent Orange and other herbicides in Vietnam." *Nature* 422, no. 6933 (2003): 681-687.

Swinney, Clare. "Declassified NZ Defense Force reports reveal chemtrail linked to outbreak of illnesses." InfoNews.co.nz, 2011. http://infonews.co.nz/news.cfm?id=62532.

Swithers, Susan E. "Artificial sweeteners produce the counterintuitive effect of inducing metabolic derangements." *Trends in Endocrinology & Metabolism* 24, no. 9 (2013): 431-441.

Taylor, Daniel. "Vaccinate the World: Gates, Rockefeller Seek Global Population Reduction." *Global Research.* September 7, 2010.

Thakkar, Vatsal G. "Diagnosing the wrong deficit." *The New York Times,* 2013. http://www.nytimes.com/2013/04/28/opinion/sunday/diagnosing-the-wrong-deficit.html?_r=0.

Trivieri, Jr., Larry. "Polyphenols: Why to eat plenty of fresh fruits and vegetables." Integrative Health Review, 2011. http://www.integrativehealthreview.com/eating-nutrition/polyphenols-why-to-eat-plenty-of-fresh-fruits-and-vegetables/.

Ukman, Jason. "CIA defends running vaccine program to find bin Laden." *The Washington Post,* 2011. http://www.washingtonpost.com/world/national-security/cia-defends-running-vaccine-program-to-find-bin-laden/2011/07/13/gIQAbLcFDI_story.html.

VaccineInjury.info. "State of health of unvaccinated children," n.d. http://www.vaccineinjury.info/results-unvaccinated/results-illnesses.html.

Vara, Christine. "Why Hepatitis B vaccine is not a lifestyle vaccine." Shot of Prevention, 2012. http://shotofprevention.com/2012/02/27/why-hepatitis-b-vaccine-is-not-a-lifestyle-vaccine/.

Whitaker, Julian, MD. "All about chelation." NaturalNews.com, 2009. http://www.naturalnews.com/027338_lead_chelation_health.html.

World Bank, The. "Data: Health expenditure, total of GDP." WorldBank.org, 2014. http://data.worldbank.org/indicator/SH.XPD.TOTL.ZS.

World Health Organization. "Electromagnetic Hypersensitivity." *Proceedings International Workshop on EMF Hypersensitivity, Prague, Czech Republic,* 2006. http://www.who.int/peh-emf/publications/reports/EHS_Proceedings_June2006.pdf.

World Health Organization (WHO). "Medicines: Rational use of medicines." WHO.int, 2010. http://www.who.int/mediacentre/factsheets/fs338/en/.

World Health Organization. "What are electromagnetic fields?" *WHO.Int,* 2014. http://www.who.int/peh-emf/about/WhatisEMF/en/index1.html.

York, Geoffrey, and Hayley Mick. "Last Ghost of the Vietnam War." *The Globe and Mail.* Toronto, ON, Canada: Phillip Crawley (2008).

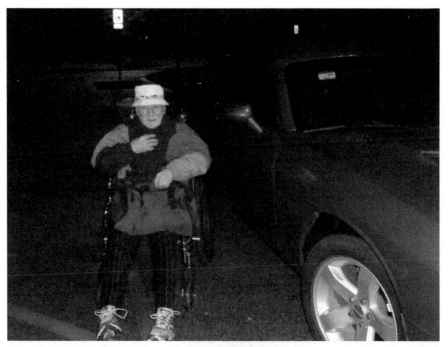

Arriving at the gym

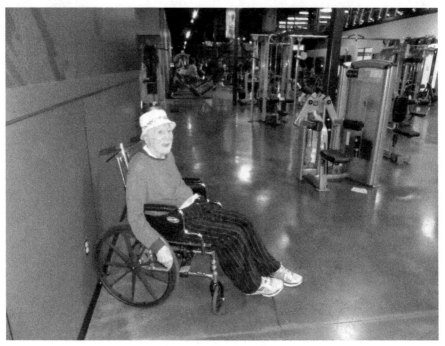

Ready to start workout

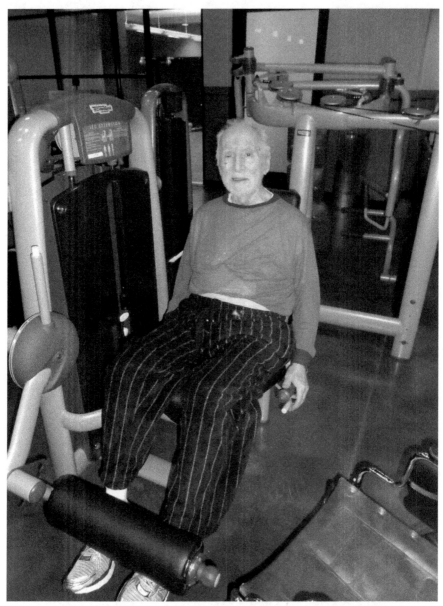

My father was an active member of Gold's Gym at age 97. This is
him doing the leg extension exercise. He would workout on a series
of 12 different machines with several sets totaling 50 repetitions
for each exercise using light weights to prevent injury.

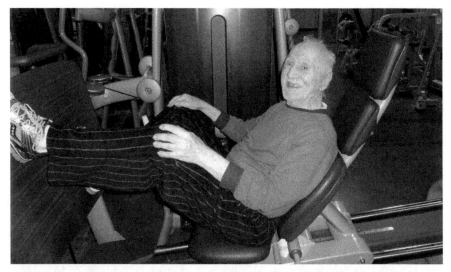

The leg press was a very important exercise as he had become disabled after a hip replacement surgery for arthritis 28 years earlier and almost died from the dangerous operation. He even had the doctor redo the operation two more times. I did not know how to use natural treatments at this time and we had a false sense of over confident and trust in conventional medicine. Finally his surgeon told my father, "Never have an operation like this again!! You almost died in recovery."

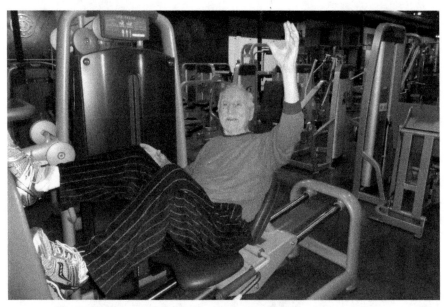

My father at age 97 doing the leg press. This machine has many handles that made it easy for my father to use without any assistance. Most gyms do not have this kind of fancy equipment

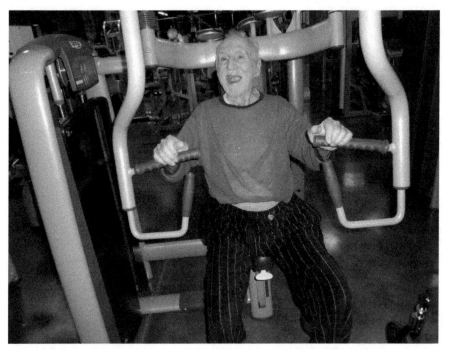

Chest Press

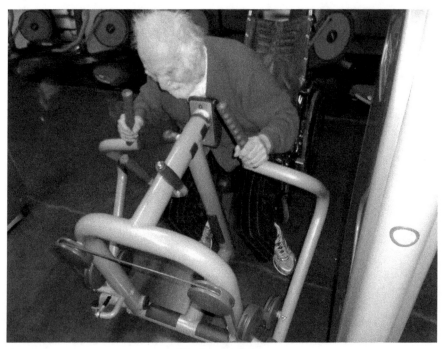

Rowing machine

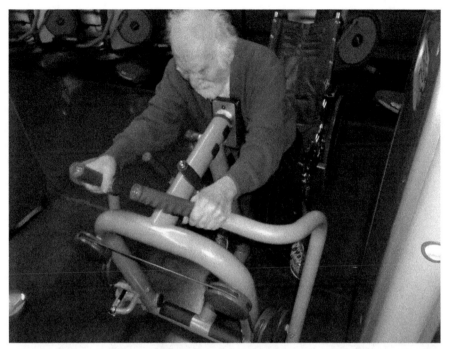

This exercise builds the back and the biceps

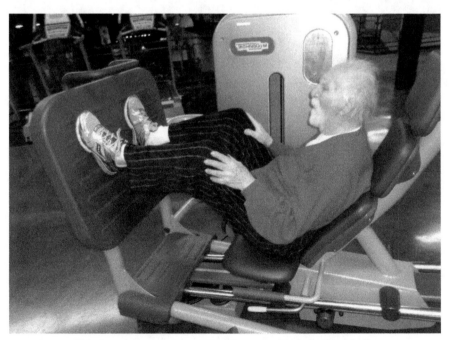

This is my father at age 97 at the gym. He is in the middle
of a set of 50 repetitions on the leg press machine

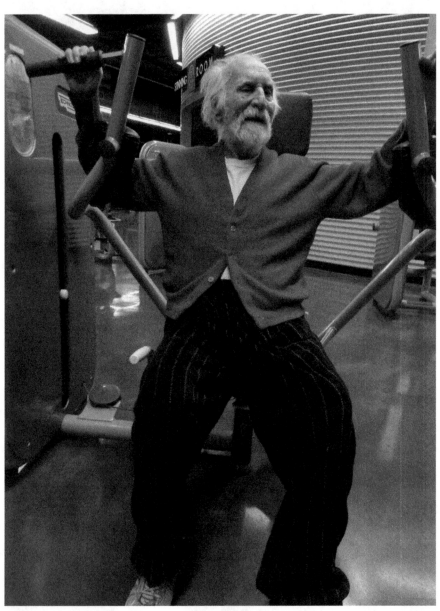

Fly machine
Exercise is part of the Anti Aging lifestyle. My father at age 97.

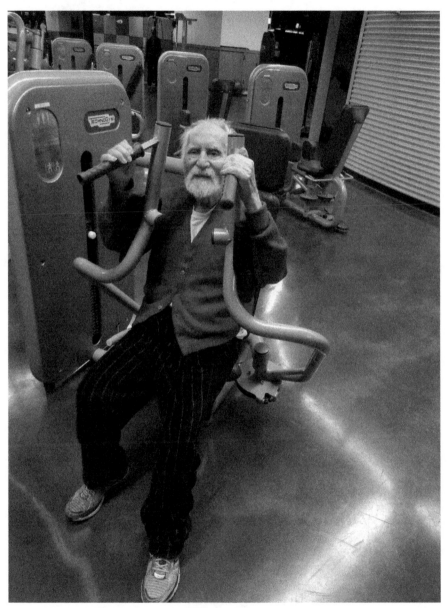

Fly machine

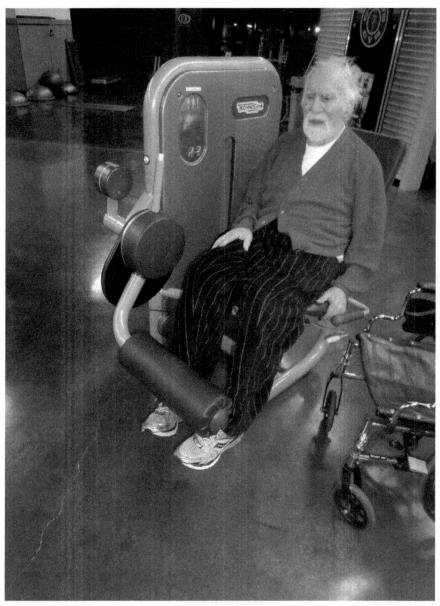

Leg Extension
We went to the gym three to five times a week for two to three hours. My father had many breaks in between each exercise. He thought of it as a way to relax.

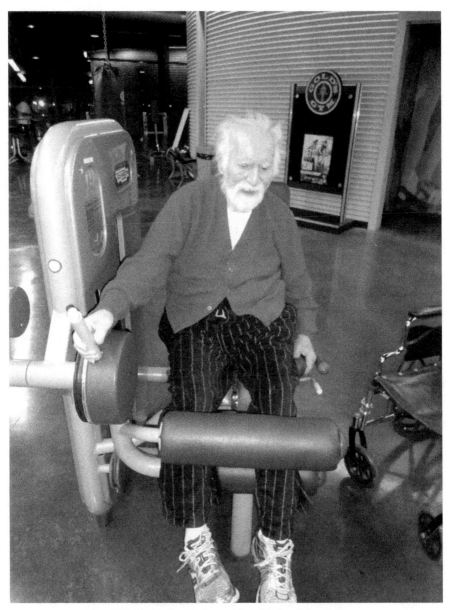

This is the leg curl exercise. Maintaining leg
strength is very important in the eldery.

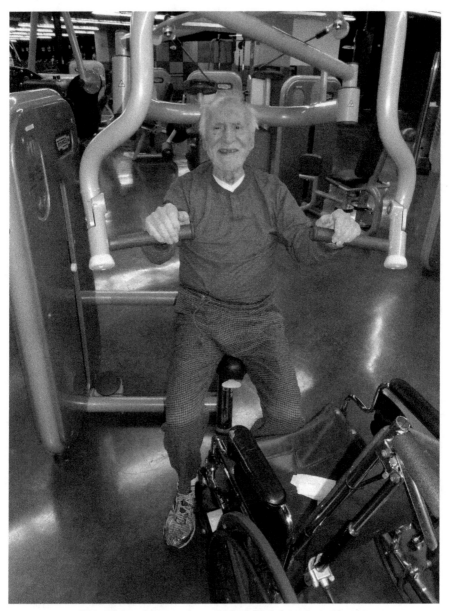

This is the chest press machine. Both leg strength and
arm strength are needed to prevent falls.

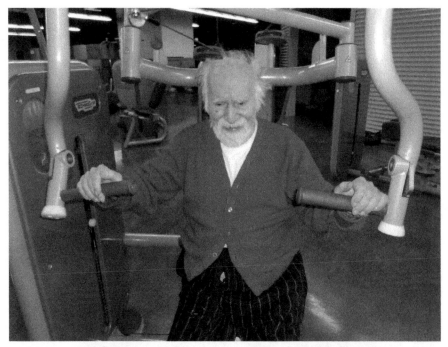

Exercise is very effective at preventing symptoms such as
depression. My father enjoyed his evenings at the gym.

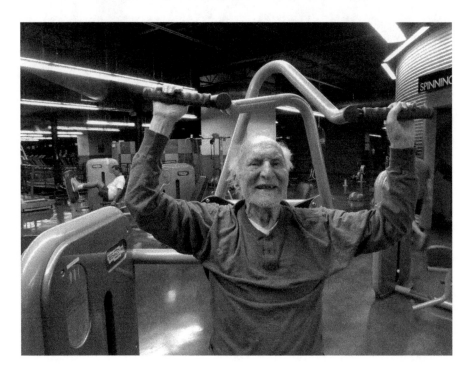

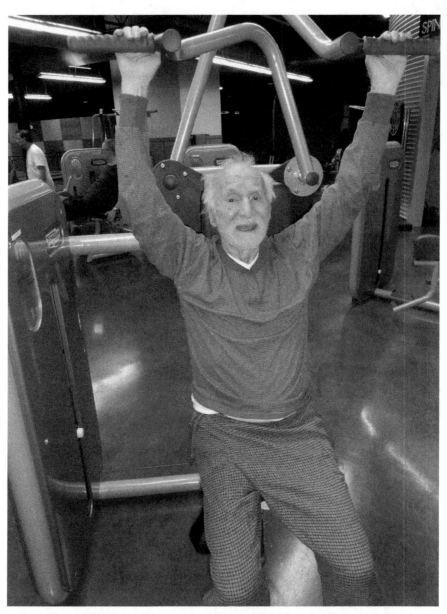

The pull down machine works the same muscles as doing chin ups.
My father always did 50 repetitions on each weight machine

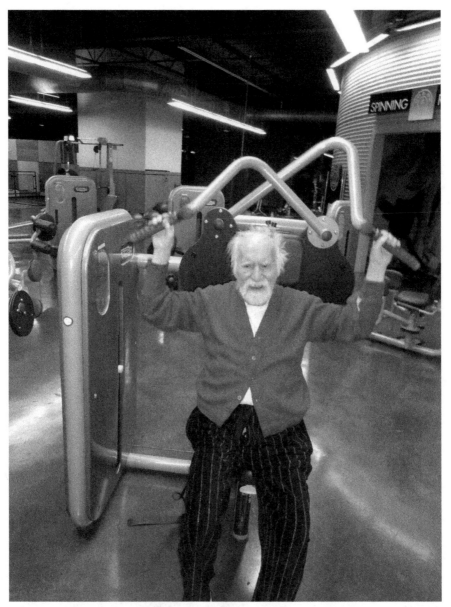
Another day at the gym.
Regular exercise is part of the Anti Aging life style

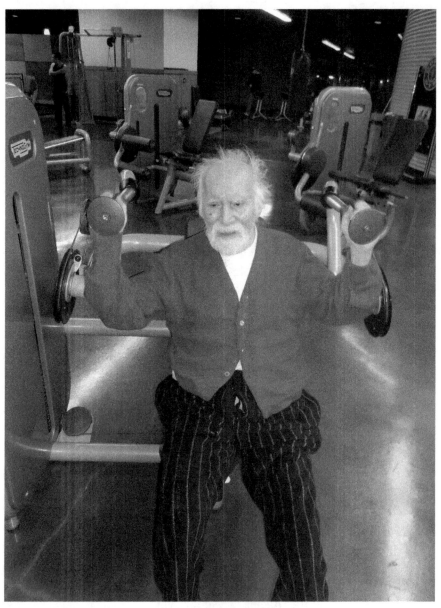

Triceps exercise

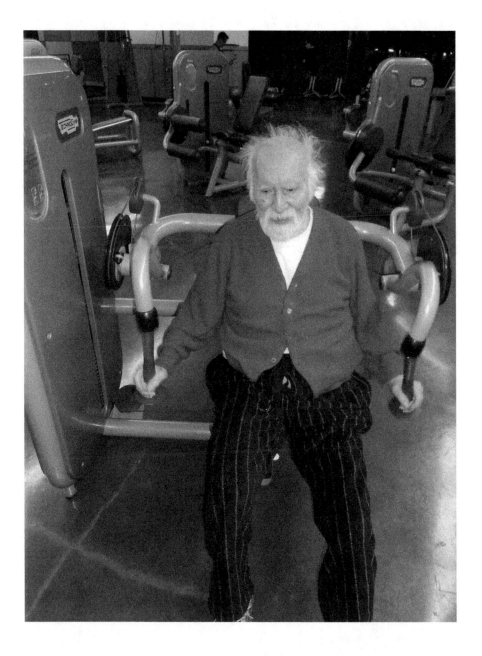

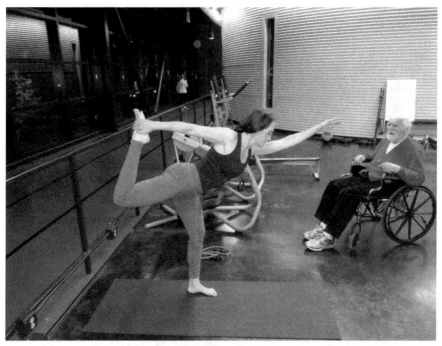

This is my 97 year old father watching his daughter, Karen age 57 at the gym

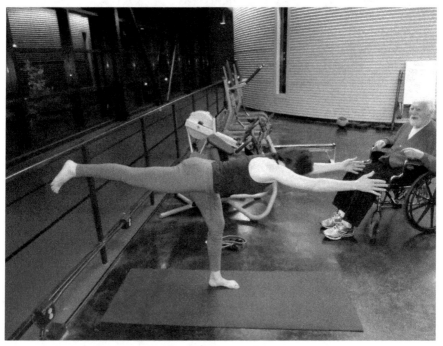

Karen and father at the gym

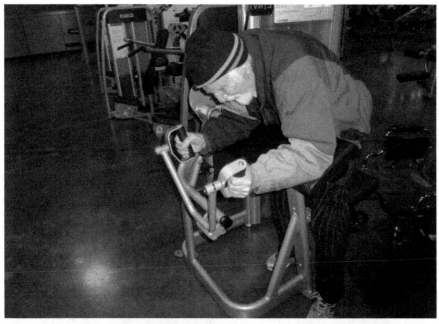

Biceps curl machine. My father liked to finish his workout with a few sets of curls.

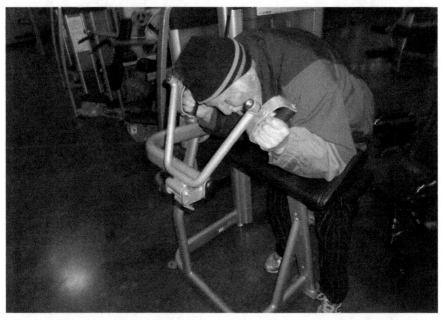

Traditional nursing home "care" of bed rest is a quick way to increase mortality and death. This is the end of a typical 2 to 3 hour day at the gym. Sometimes my father would stay another 90 minutes to take a shower. Many times we would go out to eat afterwards and then start our 50 minute trip back home.

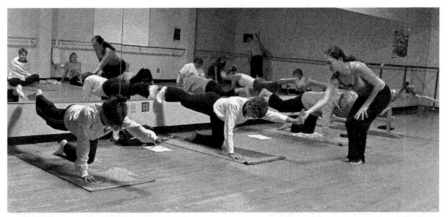

My sister Karen teaching a yoga class as part of her Anti Aging lifestyle. At age 57, she also has a healthy anti aging diet, takes numerous bio-identical hormones, chelation treatments, vitamins, herbs, Omega 3 oils, and polyphenol extracts

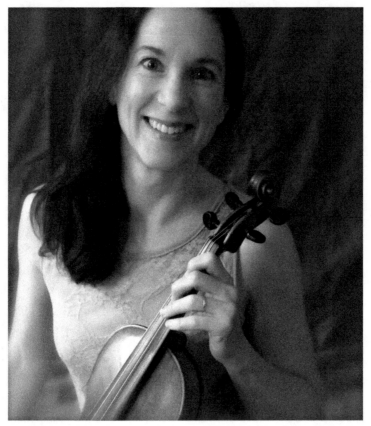

My sister with her violin. She completed a master's degree in music performance and played in professional orchestras before becoming an optometrist.

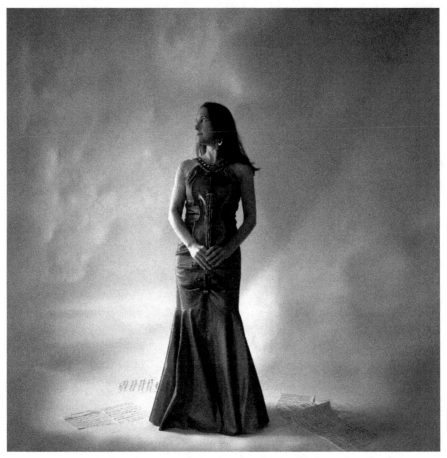
Music is well known as an effective therapy to lower stress

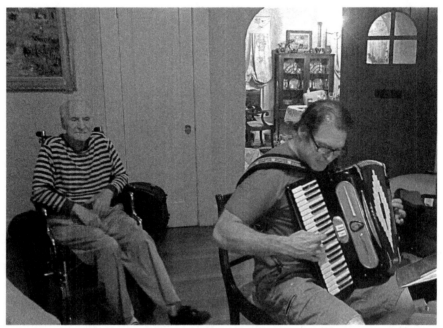

Christmas 2012
Me playing accordion with my father watching.

My father had made an amazing recovery from an automobile accident involving a speeding truck that resulted in his hospitalization in the summer of 2010 when he was 93 years old. Eventually I had to take him home "against medical advice" to speed up and make a more complete recovery. There were rumors that he would pass away in 6 months. There is an on going and unsolved mystery/crime story surrounding this freak automobile accident that is currently being investigated.

I attribute his extreme longevity and recovery not only to nutrition and exercise, but also to the fact that he was a world class musician, the world's only string bass soloist to bridge jazz, pop and classical music at a world class international level of skill. He was also an expert musician on the flute and learned to play numerous different instruments. There is enough material here for another book about his life and about exploring the relationship between health, music and longevity.

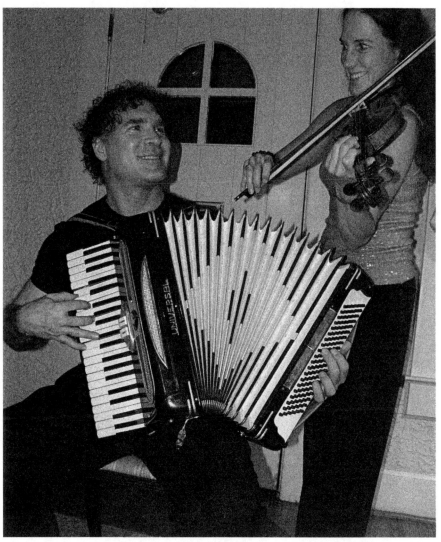

Christmas 2012
I am playing accordion with my sister on the violin Christmas 2012

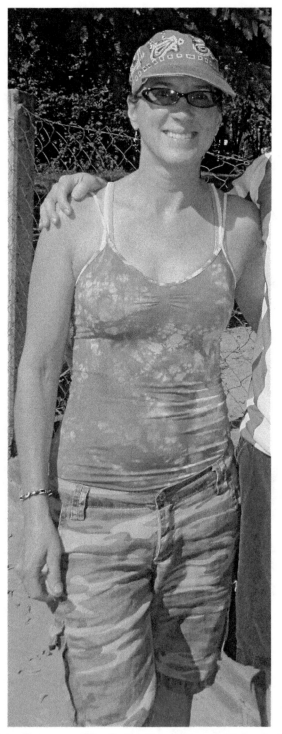

My sister Karen, age 57 enjoying the outdoors with her husband

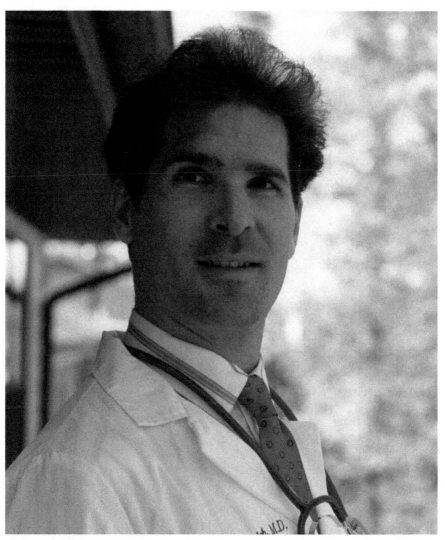

Dr. Kevin Ford age 33

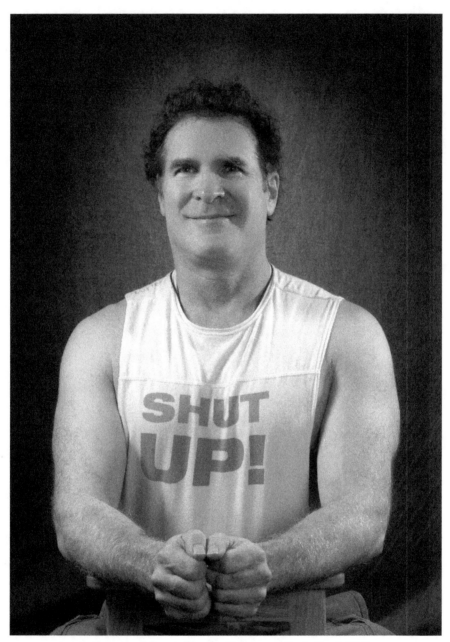

Author, musician and longevity expert, Kevin Ford, M.D.

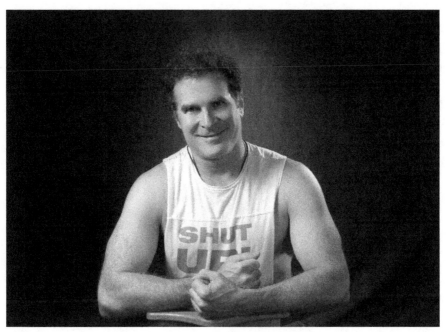

Dr. Kevin Ford age 57

ABOUT THE AUTHOR

Dr. Ford is a specialist in Anti-Aging, Regenerative, and Functional Medicine with an Advanced Fellowship Certification from the American Academy of Anti Aging Medicine. He is devoted to achieving the ultimate Anti Aging Plan.